3.00

HOW YOU CAN BEAT THE KILLER DISEASES

HOW YOU CAN BEAT THE KILLER DISEASES

HAROLD W. HARPER, M.D.

MICHAEL L. CULBERT

ARLINGTON HOUSE·PUBLISHERS
NEW ROCHELLE, NEW YORK

Manufactured in the United States of America

Library of Congress Cataloging in Publication Data

Harper, Harold W
  How you can beat the killer diseases.

  Bibliography: p.
  Includes index.
  1. Orthomolecular medicine. I. Culbert, Michael L., 1937–   joint author. II. Title [DNLM: 1. Diet—Prevention and control. 4. Metabolic diseases—Prevention and control. QU145 H294h]
RM216.H285   615'.854   77-10782
ISBN 0-87000-387-9

To all my patients who have been patient and have understood the interruptions and calls for help that I have been unable to refuse.—H.W.H.

Contents

Foreword

There was Grubbe, who first proposed to use X-ray therapy for cancer, and was excommunicated by his medical peers for so outlandish a suggestion. There was Mason, who discovered the action of penicillin before the twentieth century, and divulged his observations only to his secret diary, lest "my fellow doctors think me crazy!" There was Jenner, whose discovery of smallpox vaccine was for five years ignored by his medical society. There was Smith Ely Jelliffe, who proposed the concept of psychosomatic illness, was advised by his peers to join the Christian Science church, and died, his widow tells me, with a broken heart. There were the physicians of the British navy, who waited 50 years to act upon Lind's discovery that fresh fruit will prevent scurvy. There was the German researcher who invented the electroencephalograph, of which now familiar tool of neurology the American Medical Association remarked: "American men of medicine are too smart to fall for this type of electronic quackery." There was Semmelweiss, whose persecution is obviously not unique in medical history.

Nor have the years diluted the antagonism of medicine to innovative thinking. Feingold's discovery that food additives may initiate or aggravate hyperactivity in children was recently described by an AMA editorialist as "snake oil." Linus Pauling's proposal of orthomolecular approaches to "mental" diseases was met with booing at a meeting of the orthodox in psychiatry—in the 1960s—though Freud himself thought that chemistry would one day replace couch and conversation. It was establishment medicine that rejected the low carbohydrate reducing diet as "modern food faddism," though such diets have been used successfully for more than a century. It was orthodox medicine that labeled hypoglycemia a "nondisease"—so rare as to be nonexistent, while tens of thousands suffering from it and its Pandora's boxful of distressing symptoms went from physician to physician, only to be labeled hypochondriacs, neurotics, or even psychotics.

Orthodoxy's unwillingness to test the new is matched by its stubborn blindness to the dangers and failures of the old. Consider the cancers caused by profligate prescribing of estrogens for menopausal women, the strokes initiated by birth control pills, the irreversible brain damage and the tardive dyskinesias (involuntary fragmented movements) in schizophrenics on long-term dosage of thorazene tranquilizers. Reflect on the dismal failures with heart transplants, and the cancers derived from deliberate efforts to depress the immune mechanism of the body in an effort to avoid rejection of transplants. Remember that the successes of bypass surgery for cardiovascular disease are matched by untrumpeted (and lethal) failures. But the estrogens are still prescribed, the tranquilizer prescriptions still flow as if from a printing press, and bypass surgery is still described as the golden gift of the scalpel to suffering mankind.

Part of the resistance of orthodox medicine to change is based on an ancient axiom, solemnly passed to each generation of medical students: Be not the first to lay the old aside, nor yet the last to adopt the new. Strictly interpreted and applied, this philosophy would obviously bar all medical advances. That it does not is a tribute to the courage of medical pioneers who reject indoctrination. But how, asks the layman, can the medical establishment hold so tight a checkrein on the medical mind? After all, no one can stop a man from thinking! And this is true, but there are ways of making very difficult the translation of thoughts into action. The medical discoverer can find his hospital associations suddenly threatened or abruptly terminated. If he is practicing what his peers —by their own arbitrary definition—consider to be unorthodox medicine, he can be chastised by his medical society, and if he fails to defer to this threat, his right to practice may be suspended. If he is guilty of approaches to medicine that are too innovative—however successful—the computers of the insurance companies will balk at authorizing payment of his fees, though they will complacently allow him to be paid if his treatment is orthodox—*and* useless to the patient. If he affiliates with other rebels in medical societies too far removed from the acceptable, he will find that he cannot receive continuing medical education credits for postgraduate studies under such auspices—and without such credits, he cannot retain his right to practice. Oh, yes! there are reins, there are invisible leashes, and there are covert punishments for persistent transgressors in medicine.

Some of the opposition to innovation surfaces in the mass media, where the public is told that acupuncture invokes nothing more than the power of suggestion, which must startle the Chinese and American veterinarians who have used it successfully to treat horses and mules. Newspaper medical columns condemn herbology, though every physician uses digitalis, derived from a weed, and reserpine, found in snake root. On television, physicians assure the public that benefits from nutritional therapies are all based on spontaneous remission, when they are not a by-product of faulty diagnosis. With megavitamin therapy, these experts assure the public, it is the practitioner rather than the patient who is psychotic: why would a sane physician give vitamins to a schizophrenic who is deficient only in chlorpromazine, tofranil, or haldol? As for chelation, the FDA and the AMA unite in pronouncing it too new (it is decades old), untried (it has been used on tens of thousands of patients), ineffective (it has restored untold thousands of patients to social and vocational usefulness), and dangerous (a totally unwarranted claim when it is not explained that any medical procedure carries with it some element of danger, which in the case of chelation is infinitely smaller than that of the ineffective treatments it replaces).

I know of a 50-year-old whose heart disease (two severe attacks) and atherosclerosis were so advanced that heart surgeons, perhaps fortunately for him, refused to perform bypass surgery—he would not, they thought, survive the operation. With premature senility complicating his desperate plight, he underwent chelation, not because he believed it would help him, but because medicine had nothing more to offer. Six months later, he returned to his original physician, who looked at him in total disbelief, for he was not only totally free of symptoms, both of heart disease and senility, but appeared actually to have recaptured youth. The patient explained that he had taken chelation therapy, and ventured the surmise that, despite the physician's amazement at the benefits he had received, the doctor would not recommend the treatment for other patients. Said his physician, perhaps in

11

seriousness: "I wouldn't—but I'm going to take it myself." His philosophy resembles that of the Canadian physicians who refuse to prescribe vitamin E for their cardiac patients, but take it themselves.

At a medical convention, I chatted with a 65-year-old physician who was forced to retire from practice because of a very severe angina that followed a heart attack. He insisted that I accompany him for a brisk walk, during which we mounted a fairly steep hill. At his urging, I took his pulse when we started, and again at the top. He pointed out that his response to the effort was not that of an elderly man who had suffered heart damage, but more like that of a trained athlete. "Before chelation," he told me, "I couldn't walk upstairs without taking a nitroglycerin at the bottom, another at the top, and a rest in between. And I'm back in practice now."

When Senator Kefauver gave the Food and Drug Administration the right to judge the efficacy of drugs and vitamins, I pleaded with him not to do so. That, I urged, should be decided by the practicing physician—by the clinician, not by a government agency. Watching that agency harass physicians who prescribe Laetrile, watching it raid—and I mean *raid*— the offices of physicians who are helping their patients with chelation, I am often reminded of that conversation with the senator. I was then a Cassandra—given the gift of prophecy, with the stipulation that I should not be believed. Believe me now when I tell you that the destructive surgery of today will vanish, and the pill-pushers will surrender medicine to the biochemist, the enzymologist, and the nutritionist in medicine. And high on the gold tablets will be inscribed the names of the pioneers who resisted the pressures of their peers and government agencies—to benefit their patients.

CARLTON FREDERICKS, PH.D.
Honorary Lifetime Fellow
American Academy of Medical Preventics

12

Acknowledgments

No single person or writing team can possibly do all of the enormous tasks that must be done to complete a manuscript. Many patients have assisted with suggestions; many of our associates, physicians as well as our office staff, have made contributions too numerous to list. But one person, Bee Fletcher, has been saddled with the volumes of research, manuscript preparation, rewriting, and indexing that were necessary to accomplish the end result; to her a special thanks for her contributions.

Forbidden Medicine

In December, 1973, an 81-year-old woman suffered her ninth stroke. At the request of her family she was seen by Harold W. Harper, M.D., the physician who is one of the authors of this book. She was almost completely immobile, lying in bed, unable to communicate, unable to be understood. Her right side was paralyzed. She was using a hearing aid and still could not understand her family. She referred to her husband as her daughter, her daughter as her son-in-law and so on. She was incontinent and had had an "indwelling" catheter since her eighth stroke. She was unable to walk and unable to eat solid food. She could drink liquids only out of the left side of her mouth using a straw.

She was admitted to a Southern California hospital for a complete diagnostic workup, and as a result, Dr. Harper suggested that she undergo a form of treatment called chelation therapy, in which a chemical is administered intravenously in order to remove toxic minerals from the arteries. This therapy is being used more and more by "dissident" doctors as the treatment of choice for arteriosclerotic heart disease, but it is still essentially taboo in Establishment medicine, and the hospital refused to allow her to receive such therapy.

The woman was transferred to a nursing home where she received chelation therapy. After the third treatment the patient began to recognize the members of her family. After the fifth treatment reflexes returned to her right extremities and after the seventh she was able to leave her bed to use a bedside commode. After the twelfth treatment she was continent and the catheter was removed. She began walking with the help of attendants after the tenth treatment, and by the six-

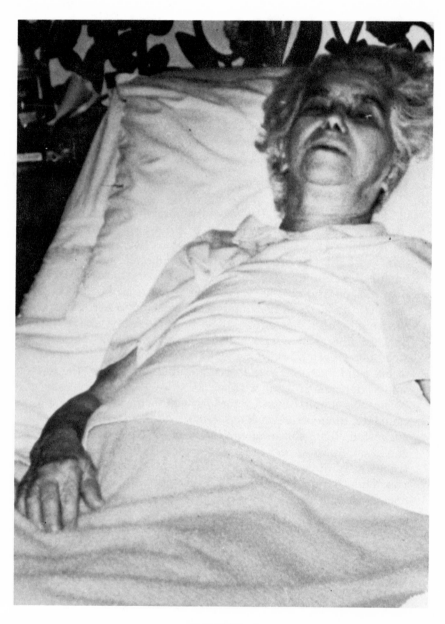

FIGURE 1

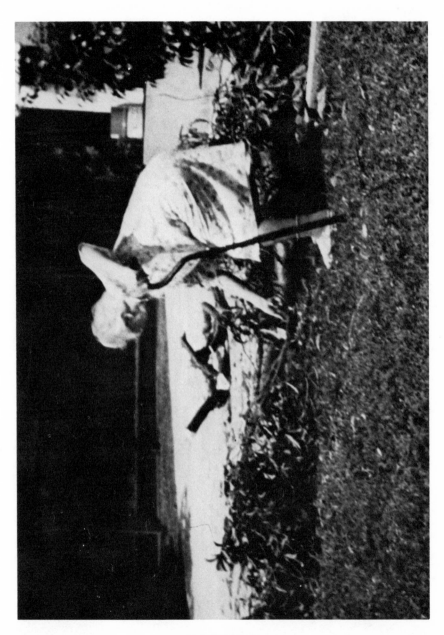

FIGURE 2

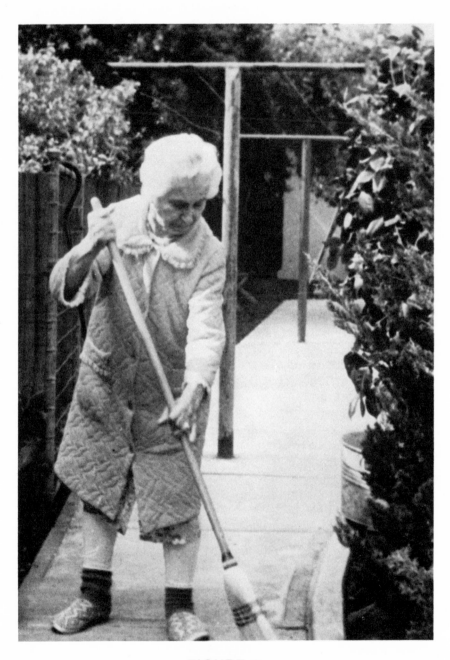

FIGURE 3

teenth she was able to walk unassisted 150 yards with a walker. By the eighteenth treatment she had doubled that distance.

The woman who was brought into the nursing home in a semicomatose state was able to walk out of that same nursing home two months later. Her progress can be seen in figures 1 through 3. In figure 1, the patient is in bed after her strokes, before receiving chelation therapy. Figures 2 and 3 were taken at her home, the former several months after beginning chelation therapy and the latter about two years later. Note that in figure 3 she does not even need a cane as she did earlier.

She and her family were able to choose an "unorthodox" therapy for one of the degenerative Killer Diseases plaguing the civilized world. The use of this treatment has involved a number of physicians in battles for their medical licenses in several states. But, as we shall see in chapter three, the alternative treatments (those not considered unorthodox) leave much to be desired. These include expensive and risky surgery, arterial dilating agents, and most often, nothing more than the careful observation of the patient by his physicians until it is time to call the mortician.

In the case described above, the previous attending physician had stated to the family that the patient would survive only two to four weeks when she was discharged from a hospital. This was two weeks before she was originally seen by Dr. Harper. Thus, although she was "sent home to die" two weeks before even being examined by Dr. Harper, she has had more than two years of active, functional life and still survives today.

Another case treated by Dr. Harper with chelation therapy is that of E. H., a 78-year-old man who was first seen in July, 1974. He and his wife reported that he had had inadequate circulation and that they had noticed a discoloration of his left leg during the preceding few months. He had difficulty walking, became short of breath on walking across a room, and could not wear normal shoes because the large toe of his left foot and the right heel showed the degenerated tissue of grossly infected gangrene. The discoloration of his left leg four inches below the knee indicated the onset of "wet" gangrene (figures 4 and 5).

Examination of the patient also showed that he had high

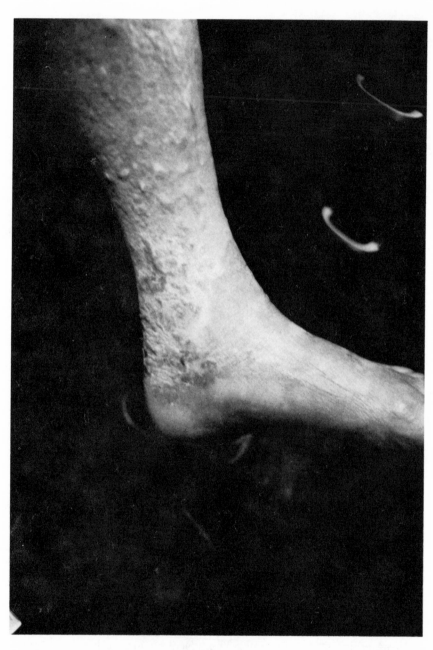

FIGURE 4

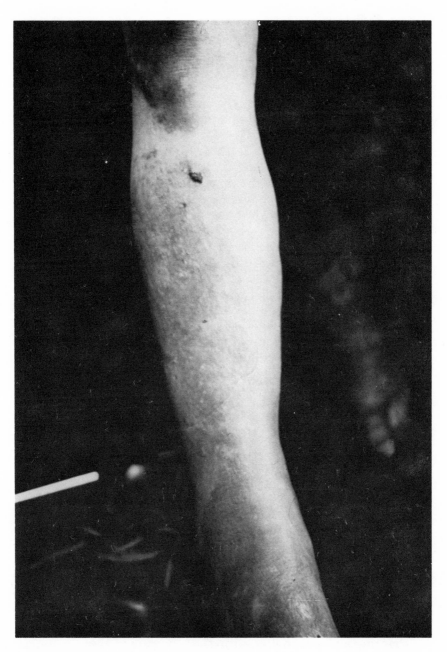

FIGURE 5

blood pressure, a marked irregularity of the heart, and fluid in the lung as a result of congestive heart failure. After proper laboratory testing, an emergency course of chelation therapy was begun five days a week for the first 21 treatments.

The normal color gradually returned to his feet and the infected gangrenous lesions began to clear as his circulation increased due to the chelating agent. When E. H. completed 40 treatments on December 7, 1974, his formerly infected leg was completely clear of any evidence of gangrene from four inches below the knee to the tip of his toes. His blood pressure was now 110 over 80, his lungs were completely clear, and he could sleep an entire night lying in a prone position without shortness of breath.

E. H. reported in December, 1974, that he was able to walk for several blocks without difficulty and without the limp and abnormal gait he had previously exhibited. He was placed on a program of a normal diet without refined carbohydrates and appropriate vitamin and mineral supplements as well as an exercise program. He was last seen as a patient on February 25, 1975. At that time he was encouraged to continue the vitamins and minerals with the diet of no refined carbohydrates and an adequate exercise program for the rest of his life.

In February, 1977, the following letter was received: "Dear Dr. Harper: Though you are not by nature bashful, you shouldn't be abashed at divulging that 'your' octogenarian legs walked ten miles easily, and they ascended Mount Hollywood. Best regards, E. H."

Figures 6 and 7 show the condition of E. H.'s legs in August, 1977. There is no sign of gangrene. (The area of dark pigmentation is skin that was less severely affected and did not slough off.)

At one point the parents of Linda G. believed they should have her committed to a mental institution. She had virtually lived in a world of her own since age 13 and was coasting through school without reading a book, alternately depressed and happy. She experimented with Far Eastern religions, tuning in and out of her surroundings, at times dreamily chanting and even hallucinating.

She remembers now that in school she was the standing joke, the girl who, at 92 pounds, tried to gain weight with a

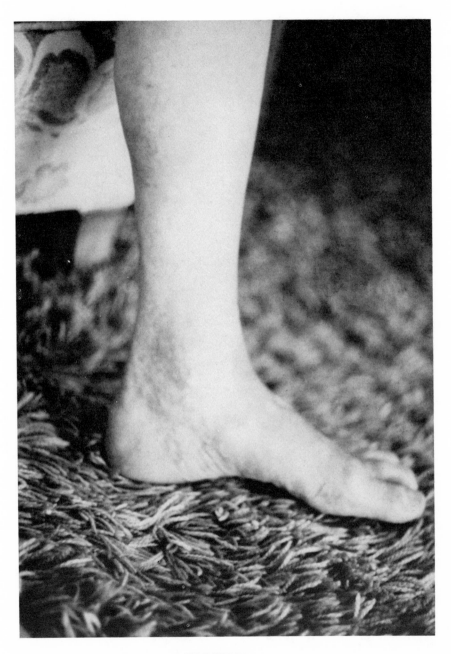

FIGURE 6

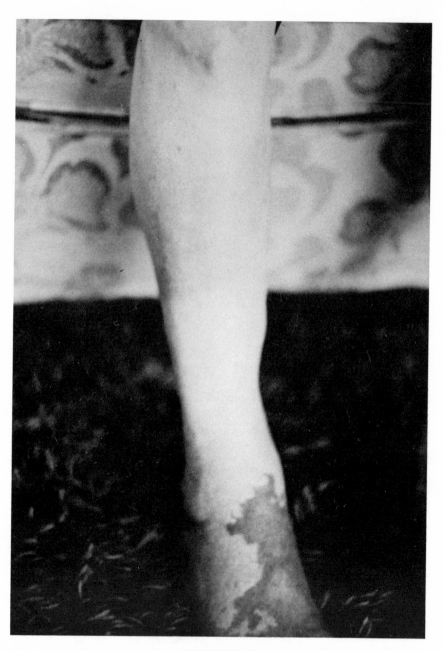

FIGURE 7

diet of five candy bars and a malted milk for lunch, and yet could not seem to gain a pound.

Linda found school boring even though on special testing programs she placed at the top of her class. She enrolled in and dropped out of four colleges before turning 21.

Then she underwent an emotional upheaval over a boy friend. Whereas before she had craved sugar constantly and was consuming up to five pounds of sugar a day (usually in the form of candy bars) without gaining weight, now she plunged into deep depression, stopped eating regularly—and began to gain weight.

It was because of her weight problem that she eventually visited Dr. Harper. By this time she was back on a regimen of "junk food" and had gained 45 pounds in two weeks.

She recalls this period in her life: "I would get up in the middle of the night, shaking and perspiring, and I had to get a cup of sugar. I didn't know what was happening. I was frightened and erratic and thought all of this had to do with emotional problems, and so did my parents."

Given a glucose tolerance test to determine how her body was handling carbohydrates, she was diagnosed as being a borderline hypoglycemic—that is, a person who has low blood sugar.

She was placed on a special diet and immediately began improving. This lasted for about one year.

Then she went through another emotional trauma and began drinking heavily. She paralleled all-day drinking with all-day consumption of sugar, eating five pounds of chocolates a day by the Christmas holidays. Once she awakened in the middle of the night with a severe craving for candy and discovered that there was none left in the house. Shaking, she began eating plain white sugar once again—and realized her problem had returned.

She returned to Dr. Harper and took another glucose tolerance test. This time she was diagnosed as having dysinsulinemia, the stage between hypoglycemia and diabetes.

That was seven years ago. At that time she went back to a strictly controlled eating plan that banned all refined carbohydrates and emphasized protein and vitamins. Within six to seven months her moods of depression vanished, and they have been absent since that time.

Now back in school as a premed student, Linda says: "It's

like being reborn. Only a hypoglycemic knows what it's like to have a hypoglycemic high followed by the lowest low. You feel like a freak, not a human being."

Hypoglycemia afflicts perhaps 30 percent or more of the American population and is the most misdiagnosed condition in medicine. Although millions of hypoglycemics are routinely diagnosed as suffering from something else and shuttled back and forth from specialist to specialist, the condition is amenable to early detection and treatment using natural, nutritional means involving the body's whole chemistry, or metabolism. Yet, the use of nutrition and vitamins in correcting disease states remains one of the least understood, let alone accepted, modalities in American medicine.

In 1976, Ray Hester, a husky linebacker with the New Orleans Saints football team, lay dying. In 1974 he had been diagnosed as having Hodgkin's disease, a form of cancer. He had gone the full route in orthodox therapy: three series of treatments with chemotherapeutic agents, followed by burning radiation. Then he received what amounted to a death warrant.

Approximately 5 percent of cancer patients who undergo cobalt radiation treatment also come down with another form of cancer as a result: leukemia. "I was one of the 5 percent," he recalls, "so now I had both Hodgkin's and leukemia."

For two months Ray lived in a sterile environment inside a plastic tent in a hospital, completely cut off from normal surroundings, so that he would not be exposed to infection of any kind. By this time he was virtually living on donated blood since his capacity to produce white blood cells had all but been eliminated.

In desperation, his physicians offered to use him as a guinea pig for the testing of a new drug in hopes that this might prolong his life. Before this new treatment was to begin he was released from the hospital and told to return in two weeks.

But during this hiatus he learned through a friend about the metabolic and nutritional treatment of cancer, including the use of Laetrile, or vitamin B_{17}, along with other vitamins and enzymes. He also learned about the imagery and self-hypnosis techniques of mentally attacking cancer that were pioneered by Dr. Carl O. Simonton of Dallas.

The use of Laetrile, the processed form of vitamin B_{17}, has never been made illegal by law, but it has been banned from *interstate* shipment and sale by internal regulations of the United States Food and Drug Administration (FDA). In spite of this restriction, Hester was able to make a "Laetrile connection" and receive the substance. He told us in December, 1976, when we met him: "Under Laetrile my blood count doubled in five days. The signs of leukemia were gone in 20 days."

Hester had taken up to 4.5 grams of Laetrile a day at one point, as well as using enzymes and other vitamins and adhering strictly to a diet of fresh fruits and vegetables and their juices and abstaining from all animal protein.

While at one time he had been given a day at a time to live, Ray Hester was pronounced free of all cancerous activity in September, 1976. Subsequent hospital checkups by amazed orthodox physicians continue to confirm his turnaround.

"I can't say it's been just the imagery or the Laetrile or the diet and enzymes, but something has worked," Hester told us.

The former football player beat most of the odds—but died in the summer of 1977, more than a year and half after he was given up for dead.

The case of Alycia Buttons, wife of comedian Red Buttons, came to light in 1973. She had been diagnosed as a "terminal" throat cancer patient, but she brought her cancer under control through Laetrile and a program of enzyme therapy, vitamins, minerals and dietary change at the West German clinic of Dr. Hans Nieper. Her malignancy is still under control at the time this is being written.

Her much publicized case underscored the plight of other terminal American cancer patients. They are told that orthodox modalities can do nothing for them and they also discover that the use of Laetrile is indirectly banned in the United States. Thus, they are forced either to flee their own country and seek Laetrile-metabolic therapy in other countries or to try to find one of the few physicians in the United States who are using the program in defiance of the regulations.

Equally impressive is the case of Pam McDaniel, a High Point, North Carolina, theology student who in March, 1975, was diagnosed as having terminal, metastasized osteosarcoma (bone cancer) in both legs; moreover, the disease had spread to other parts of her body.

"I was told not to expect to see Christmas 1975," Miss Mc-

Daniel said. "I was using crutches and my legs were locking. The doctors were honest enough to tell me it would be useless to try chemotherapy and they also said radiation would burn everything else before it even got to the leg bones."

In great pain, Pam McDaniel saw 21 doctors before there was a consensus that the treatment she should receive was surgery in which she would lose part or all of both her legs. Furthermore, her physicians warned that even then there was a fifty-fifty chance that she would be paralyzed below the hips.

But before the surgery was performed, Pam learned about Laetrile and the metabolic management of cancer. She took 20 cc (6 grams) of Laetrile intravenously every day for 43 days, then 20 cc every third day, and then injections and tablets on alternating days while following the special metabolic program diet.

Her former doctors were stunned. They had not believed she could live through 1975, and now, during 1976, she had no trace of cancer at all.

Pam McDaniel started on the Laetrile program after having been regarded as terminally ill. No other treatment was given. In spite of the results, the doctor who treated her later came under fire from his state medical board because he was using a substance held to be an "unproven remedy" by orthodox American medicine.

While this is being written it is too early to class the McDaniel—and many other—cases as "cures," but they are, at least, short-term "controls" of cancer. Such cancer victims have already beaten tremendous odds by using the unorthodox approach.

Throughout the country, physicians are being pressured, and at times punished, for their use of Laetrile and its related therapy in the management of cancer. In California several have been arrested, and members of an "international Laetrile smuggling ring" providing United States physicians and their patients with Mexican Laetrile were convicted by the federal government in a three-month-long trial in San Diego, California, which cost taxpayers millions of dollars.

Yet, in 27 other countries Laetrile is legal—or at least not officially interefered with—and a large number of case histories of cancer victims reporting a wide range of benefits through use of the full Laetrile program is being built.

Cancer now strikes one out of every four Americans and kills one out of every six. It is the major killer of children and the second major killer of adults in the United States. Yet physicians who use Laetrile and other nontoxic, potentially inexpensive, and simple modalities in the treatment of cancer are routinely persecuted.

Even worse is the situation with arteriosclerotic vascular disease, "heart disease," which is responsible for one out of every two fatalities in the United States every year. While it is far and away the biggest of the Killer Diseases, the crisis medicine with which it is treated has made no appreciable dent in either preventing or curing the heart disease catastrophe.

The United States is now stalked not by the specter of infectious diseases and parasites but by the degenerative Killer Diseases. Babies are born with arthritis, young adults have significant arteriosclerosis at age 22, children are victims of leukemia, teenagers develop cancer, and heart disease and strokes strike people in their thirties and forties. This is the tragic health scene in the United States and, indeed, in most of the Western world, where *manmade* diseases are the order of the day. And at the same time there is a rapidly proliferating "health-care delivery industry" that is eating up more than $140 billion in private and public funds each year in futile attempts to control these Killer Diseases.

While the nation gets sicker, not healthier, *natural* approaches to prevention and healing are getting the bum's rush.

ONE

Man on the Way to Self-Extinction

PERVERTING OUR HERITAGE

In the beginning, man was insignificant to the scheme of things. The ecosystem that is planet earth worked with clock-like precision, with plants, animals, air, and water interdependent and fueling the great cycle of life.

Eventually, however, man came to control the earth. He took what he wanted from the land for food and shelter and discarded what he did not need. In terms of total geological time man has been present on earth for little more than an instant, yet in that instant he has effected changes that have decisively upset the interlocking natural clockwork that is his heritage.

As man has progressed—if moving from a nomadic, tribal existence to an agrarian society and then to a highly technological, urban environment can be called progress—he has left a permanent mark on the planet.

Lead concentration in the Greenland ice cap, for example, has increased 1,200 percent in the last 125 years and 400 percent in the last 25 years. The measurements were made by boring deep into the ice that formed over 100 years ago and then comparing the lead concentrations in that ice to those present in the ice today. The important question is: What will the lead concentration become in the *next* 25 years?

Lead is, of course, one of the major toxic chemicals with which civilized man is killing himself and poisoning his environment. In one of the most polluted areas on earth, the Los Angeles basin, some 30,000 pounds of lead are poured into the air *daily,* creating a lead concentration in the air that is 50 times higher than that for rural areas and 5,000 times what would be present if man had never discovered the automobile. And even within Los Angeles the concentration of lead in the air varies depending on where you are located: it is increased 50 percent if you are within five blocks of a freeway or two blocks of a major thoroughfare.

In 1972, Swiss researchers found that of 232 adults living in the immediate vicinity of a major highway, 25 of them (11 percent) had died of cancer during the period between 1959 and 1970. This was nine times more than had died of cancer in a comparable "traffic-free" region.

Of the 25 who died, 22 had lived in the area near the highway for at least 10 years. Subjective complaints such as fatigue, headaches, stomach and intestinal disorders, and depression were heard during the test period from those living in this area.

Forty-seven of the residents of this area had received chelation therapy as treatment for lead poisoning. The average number of treatments was 10, although only one or two treatments were given in a few cases. Of the group that had been treated with chelation therapy only one person died of cancer during the years between 1959 and 1970. During this same period, 24 of the 185 residents who did not receive chelation therapy died of cancer, an incidence of 12.9 percent.

But lead is not, of course, the only toxic pollutant in the air we breathe. Each year, in the United States alone, an estimated 200 million tons of pollutants are spewed into the air. These include such harmful gases as sulfur and nitrogen oxides, carbon monoxide and ozone, and particles of solid matter such as asbestos, heavy metals and tar. All of these are dumped into the atmosphere over North America every year by an expanding technological society that seems to consider the surrounding air as a refuse dump.

The toxic chemicals are not only found in the air, but also in the ground, having been drained from the great industrial plants to pollute our streams and oceans and to poison the wildlife, some of which we later consume. The major technological centers in the United States are clustered on both coasts, but their toxic wastes are carried inland by prevailing winds to pollute the areas where our food is grown. And, as if that were not bad enough, more than a thousand pesticides, fungicides, and weed killers are sprayed on our farmlands *in-*

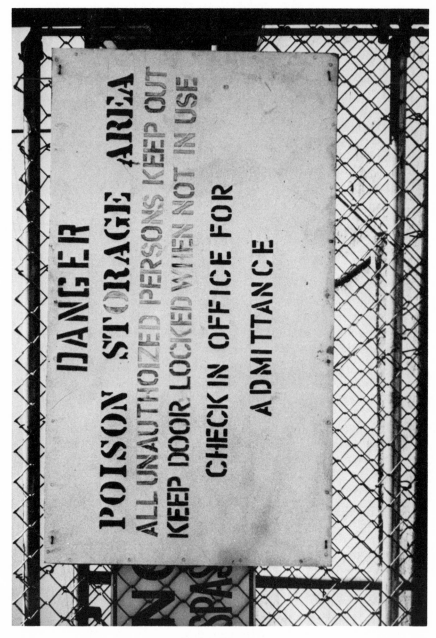

FIGURE 8

tentionally. Figure 8 shows the sign posted on a fence that encloses cropdusters and stored chemicals to be sprayed on crops. These chemicals are poisons and their toxic wastes pollute not only the crops we eat but also the animals that graze on the land, thereby contaminating the animals themselves. Our bodies become contaminated by eating both the contaminated crops and the contaminated animals.

The water we drink contains all manner of pesticides, detergents, "optical brighteners," chemical salts, fertilizers, human and animal excrement, residues of heavy toxic metals, dangerous chemicals, and even radioactive wastes. Only in the past few years has there been a growing awareness of the perils inherent in our drinking water, laden as it is with unfiltered chemicals, many of them poisonous and many of them suspected of helping to induce cancer. Analyses of the water supplies of our large cities have shown that not a single one of them is free of every one of the chemicals known to cause cancer in animals.

Attention has also been given to the problems of air pollution, although little that has been done has drastically reduced this pollution. But almost no attention has been given to the most important type of pollution—that of our food supply.

Even worse than what man has done to the balance of nature is what he has done to his body through the foods that he eats. The central thesis of this book is that proper cell metabolism, the means by which cells remain normal and healthy and thus constitute a healthy and normal living organism, requires the right amount of the right nutrients at the right time delivered to the right place—and that tampering with this interplay is the cause of degenerative disease. The wholesale tampering with natural nutrition has triggered the modern plagues of mankind, the degenerative Killer Diseases, which are the maladies caused not by bacteria, viruses and parasites, but by the continual ingestion of unnatural foods.

It is the second major thesis of this book that nothing short of major changes in lifestyle and eating habits and a return to biological sanity in food production and processing can stop or delay the widespread destruction of "civilized" people through their food supply.

THE FOOD POLLUTERS

Since 1958 the Food and Drug Administration has approved the use of more than 3,000 food additives as "Generally Recognized As Safe" and placed them on the official GRAS list. But the actual number of chemicals that go into denaturalizing our food is not known, and estimates vary widely. Some claim it is as high as 10,000. Over half of these additives are added simply to flavor, emulsify, color, buffer, thicken, or stabilize—in other words, to entice us to buy more so the food processing company will make a larger profit. Otherwise, the additives are entirely unnecessary. These chemicals and the ones used in the actual processing turn natural foods into adulterated simulations devoid of most of their nutrients, artificially colored and padded with preservatives, bleaches, texture enhancers, dough conditioners, and a large variety of other things.

In 1955 an estimated 419 million pounds of additives went into our food supply; today over a billion pounds costing over $500 million are added. Americans are consuming five pounds *per capita* of these additives each year in addition to an average of over 120 pounds of sugar, which, as we shall see, is also a major contributor to degenerative disease.

Vitamins and other natural nutrients in foods are lost through processing. The mere act of cooking will remove more than half the vitamins, and the various freezing and canning processes strip foods even further, so that by the time they reach the table they may have had removed all but trace amounts of the nutrients our bodies must have to maintain a healthy state. Thus, what most of us eat are foods loaded with preservatives, additives and calories and that lack adequate vitamins and minerals.

All that seems necessary for the success of a fast-food operation is to provide ample refined carbohydrates. The nation's major hamburger production chain, McDonalds, proudly proclaims that it has sold 22 *billion* hamburgers—or about 100 for every man, woman, and child in the United States. By the time you read this, that figure will almost certainly have passed 25 billion. This fast-food chain has thousands of sites throughout the length and breadth of the country to provide

34

nutritionless white bread containing starch and refined sugar along with more carbohydrates in the form of french fries, milkshakes, soft drinks, and desserts.

The major addiction problem in the United States and, to a large extent, in the Western world, has nothing to do with opiates, uppers or downers, or even alcohol or tobacco. The number one addiction today is to sugar—either in the form of sucrose (refined white sugar), lactose (from milk), fructose (from fruit), maltose (from malt), or glucose (dextrose).

For most of us, sugar addiction begins in the womb when our mothers consume sugar, in all its forms, while "eating for two." This virtually guarantees the addiction of the child and sets the stage for a lifelong "habit." And to satisfy this need there is a "pusher" on every corner—or even in the middle of the block. Sugar is the major ingredient in the empty-calorie junk foods that pollute the American marketplace and dinner table today. One of the nation's largest doughnut chains is now open 24 hours a day to provide not only sugar and starch at any time of day or night, but also the caffeine to go with it.

Sugar is consumed in literally thousands of ways in a variety of food products whose number increases yearly. Few people are aware that it is added to a whole variety of "nonsweet" foods including mayonnaise, catsup, salad dressings, TV dinners, canned and frozen vegetables, gelatin desserts, and cereals. Look at the label of any processed food. The chances are overwhelming that you will see sugar and/or one of its various forms listed as an ingredient.

Sometimes food processors do not like to use the word sugar, so instead they use sucrose, dextrose, dextrin, corn syrup, corn sweetener, honey, molasses, turbo sugar, lactose, maltose, or fructose. The name really does not matter, for each of these has the same effect on the body. Turbo sugar, for example, is simply sugar from which the fluid has been removed. This is usually the state in which it is shipped from Hawaii to California for its final processing. Turbo sugar differs from refined sugar only in that it has less liquid content and usually contains a fair amount of rat excrement that it picks up from the ships' holds while in transit. It is, therefore, just as damaging to the body as other forms of sugar, all of which are major contributing factors in the development of such disease states as hypoglycemia, diabetes, arteriosclerosis, cancer, gastro-intestinal disorders, and even mental illness.

Sugar itself contains none of the vitamins and minerals or other nutrients that our bodies need (hence the label "empty calories"), and not only supplies no nutrients, but depletes some of those already present in our bodies that are needed for other purposes.

The deleterious effects of sugar can also be seen in the following statistics. On the basis of per capita consumption, the three largest users of sugar are the United States, Great Britain, and Denmark. These same three countries are the only three industrial nations whose citizens have had no increase in their life expectancy since 1958.

The amount of sugar contained in processed foods is colossal. A little investigation in any supermarket shows that for most foods our only choices are between highly sugared products and only partly sugared products. It does not take long to see how easy it is for Americans to consume an average of over 120 pounds per person of sugar every year. We consume it in virtually everything we eat, with the exception of fresh fruits, vegetables, and meats. Anything that comes in a bottle, can, box, or other container is likely to contain a large amount of sugar.

While the exact amount of sugar in any particular product cannot be learned from reading labels, the position of an ingredient on the list does tell a great deal. By law, the list of ingredients must begin with the one that is present in the largest quantity by weight, with the remaining ingredients listed in descending order on the basis of weight. Thus, for example, a food like raspberry Jello, which lists its ingredients as sugar, gelatin, ascorbic acid, sodium nitrate, artificial flavor, and artificial color, has more sugar than gelatin, more gelatin than ascorbic acid, more ascorbic acid than sodium nitrate, and so on.

In addition to the sugar, there are other harmful ingredients in this particular product. Sodium nitrate is commonly used as a preservative in ham, bacon, luncheon meats, and smoked meats and fish. Nitrates and nitrites can combine in the body with other chemicals to form nitrosamine, a known carcinogenic—that is, a cancer-causer.

When "artificial flavor" and "artificial color" are listed as ingredients, it is impossible to know their exact composition.

In cases like this where the ingredients are not clearly spelled out, it is reasonable to assume that there is a reason why and that the chances are very high that you would be better off keeping these "unknown quantities" on the outside rather than the inside of your body.

The point here is not to attack raspberry Jello. There are many, many other products that are just as bad for you, if not worse.

Virtually all baby foods contain sugar. Many baby food companies refuse to tell us how much sugar their products do contain, but one independent consumer group has indicated that some baby foods contain as much as 40 percent sugar! Even the new, highly publicized "natural" baby foods are advertised as having no salt and *less* sugar. If they can remove all the salt, why not remove all the sugar, an ingredient that has many negative effects and no positive ones—except in the pocketbooks of the producers? Sugar is one of the cheapest ingredients used in processed foods, and most companies would hate to have to replace it with a more expensive one. One of the primary reasons it is included is to please the taste of the mother who buys the product and is already addicted to sugar. Thus the baby also becomes another victim of sugar addiction.

As we have already indicated, sugar is an ingredient in many products that we normally consider nonsweet. It is the fifth ingredient listed in Kraft Mayonnaise, the third ingredient listed in Heinz Tomato Ketchup, the third ingredient in chicken bouillon, the sixth and ninth ingredients listed in Lipton Onion Soup Mix, and so on ad infinitum. Even a frozen turkey dinner containing turkey with giblet gravy, dressing, mashed potatoes, and carrots and peas has *three* sources of sugar.

Furthermore, "diet foods" are no exception to this sugar extravaganza. Sugar is the *second* ingredient listed in Figurines, advertised as "The Crunchy Diet Meal."

The breakfast-food section of your supermarket is even more disastrous, from a nutritional point of view, than other sections. For example, Carnation Instant Breakfast is advertised as being for the person on the run who, with a few gulps of this product, can get a nutritious meal. The label tells us that the first and eighth ingredients are sugar.

Another breakfast drink, Tang, the "breakfast drink of the

astronauts," has sugar as its main ingredient. Of course, a few vitamins and artificial flavoring are also thrown in so we feel that we are getting something nutritious.

The advertisements for cereals are some of the most misleading of any of those for food products. For example, Kellogg's Product 19 says it is "the high-nutrition cereal." Ads for Special K assert that it is "serious nutrition for weight-conscious adults." Cocoa Puffs is advertised as "delicious and nutritious." Trix claims to be "fortified with eight essential vitamins and iron." Close inspection of the labels on these and other cereal products reveals that all have a high sugar content and that a large portion of the vitamins claimed actually comes from the milk that one adds to these cereals.

In addition, despite the fact that the United States is the largest grain producer in the world, we process these grains until we have removed the bran and the germ, which are the parts most filled with vitamins and minerals, and we "polish" rice until we have removed the majority of the minerals it once contained. This denuded material is then puffed, toasted, and sugar-coated, and promoted as "nutritious."

These same processed grains are used in making white flour which in turn is used in making bread, pastries, and so on. Of course, a few vitamins and minerals are returned to the flour so that it can be called "enriched," but this does not help very much: 22 different vitamins, minerals, and amino acids are removed and only 4 are returned.

Dr. Joe Nichols describes the process this way:

> Suppose a mugger ordered you at gunpoint to strip down to your birthday suit, giving up clothing, shoes, underwear, wallet, credit cards, jewelry—everything you possess. Then, should the thief take pity on you and return your wedding band, your socks, and perhaps your topcoat to cover your nakedness so you could get home, you might feel "enriched," but I doubt it. That's the equivalent of what's taking place in the food industry. First they strip away everything of value—then they put back a token selection of necessities and convince everyone they've been "enriched" by the process.

Since the body rapidly converts refined white flour into sugar, it is evident that white flour, even when enriched, joins sugar as a cause par excellence of degenerative disease in man. Products that contain both sugar and enriched white flour are simply doubly harmful.

The snack foods with the funny names like Ding Dongs and Twinkies afford relatively inexpensive ways to ingest large amounts of sugar and white flour, in spite of the fact that the ads suggest that they are some of the best foods you can provide for your children. The line used is: "You can't skimp when it comes to your children." Obviously, such a statement is intended to make you feel guilty if you give your children anything else.

And what about "the staff of life"? Consider, for example, Wonder Bread, which at one time was advertised as building "strong bodies twelve ways." What we were not told was that it can destroy strong bodies with two of its major ingredients: enriched flour and corn sweetener. And some of the other ingredients are not so wonderful for man either. Dough conditioners, for example, are included to make the bread stay fresh longer, to increase shelf life, and to discourage insects from eating it. The obvious question we should ask is: If insects won't eat it, should we?

After one has eaten enough of these refined, unnatural foods, discomfort often occurs in the form of stomach pains, gas, constipation, heartburn, and headaches, and instead of eliminating their cause we simply "treat" the symptoms. More often than not these "treatments" contain chemicals that further pollute our bodies. Most over-the-counter pain relievers, for example, contain caffeine, which is a habituating stimulant intimately linked to the problem of low blood sugar, as we will see in chapter two.

The nervousness, fatigue, dizziness and insomnia caused by caffeine and foods polluted by refined carbohydrates, as well as by polluted air and water, lead many Americans to want something stronger than over-the-counter drugs. Valium is one of the most popular of all medications not only because people request it from their physicians, but also because it takes far less time for a physician to write a prescription for it (about 30 seconds) than to attempt to find and correct the cause of the patient's symptoms.

In 1974, there were 59.5 *million* prescriptions for Valium written in the United States alone, with an average prescription being for between 50 and 100 tablets. That is a considerable amount of "tranquilizing," even in our polluted, stress-causing environment. One might conclude that for the most part we are a tranquilized society awaiting death.

39

CONFLICTS OF INTEREST

There are very few nutrition experts in America, and the few we have are frequently on the payroll of—or have research sponsored by—those in the food processing or pharmaceutical industries.

The Department of Nutrition at the Harvard University School of Public Health is usually considered to be the last word in nutritional education, wisdom, and research in this country. Yet, the department has accepted millions of dollars in grants from General Foods, Kellogg, Nabisco, the Sugar Association, and the International Sugar Foundation. Individual members of the department are also involved in situations which might be considered "conflicts of interest." Professor of Nutrition Frederick Stare, for example, is a consultant to the pharmaceutical and sugar industries as well as a member of the Continental Can Company board of directors.

In 1976, a consumer study group called the Center for Science in the Public Interest, along with Representative Benjamin Rosenthal, accused eminent American nutritionists of having "traded their independence for the food industry's favors." The center's study, *Feeding at the Company Trough,* points out how most nutritionists who make public analyses of consumer problems either are on the boards of food companies or have other ties with them. Dr. Michael Jacobson, the group's codirector, said: "One can only come to the conclusion that industry grants, consulting fees, and directorships are muzzling, if not prostituting, nutrition and food-science professors."

This should be kept in mind when you hear or read that the United States has the most nutritious food supply in the world and that Americans are getting a "balanced diet."

Those who turn to government as the way to keep giant food processors straight should be aware that the monitoring Food and Drug Administration is among the most scandal-ridden of federal agencies. Time and again it has been shown to be influenced, and at times controlled, by both the food processors and the international drug monopolies, those purveyors of drugs and medicines aimed quite frequently at the symptoms caused by food pollution. In 1976, for example, it was found that some 150 officers of the FDA improperly held stock in the drug companies their agency is supposed to be monitoring.

Dr. John O. Nestor, a pediatrician with the FDA, is among the FDA employees who have spoken out on the pachydermal awkwardness and slowness of the regulatory agency. He told Senate investigators in 1963 that the FDA worked too closely with the big drug companies to be objective. By 1975 he was prominently featured in a 906-page, $196,000 report issued by the then FDA Commissioner Alexander Schmidt in an attempt to defend the agency against yet another Senate probe. Dr. Nestor dismissed the report as a "whitewash," and added: "They still refuse to assign me work; most of the time I do nothing, even though I make $38,000 a year."

Anyone who believes he will be at his nutritional best by consuming foods that have the U. S. Department of Agriculture's "recommended daily allowance" (RDA) or the "minimum daily requirement" (MDR) of vitamins has been grossly misled—probably by the statements made by the FDA and the American Medical Association. There cannot be a *single* RDA or MDR that is appropriate for different individuals. In fact, these alleged recommended minimal levels are not based on individual metabolisms at all, but on what the Food and Nutrition Board calls the "reference man and woman"—a person of "normal" height and weight, living in a temperate climate and doing temperate things who is 22 years old. In other words, there are very few people in the United States to whom these standards apply.

Senator William Proxmire wrote in *Let's Live* about these "official" levels: "At best the RDAs are only a 'recommended' allowance at antediluvian levels designed to prevent terrible disease. At worst, they are based on conflicts of interest and self-serving views of certain parts of the food industry. Almost never are they provided at levels to provide for optimum health and nutrition." Of the Food and Nutritional Board, Proxmire wrote: "It is both the creature of the food industry and heavily influenced by the food industry. It is in the narrow economic interest of the industry to establish low official RDAs," so that its products will appear to be more nutritious.

In 1976, Senator Proxmire told Congress:

The Food and Drug Administration proposal to regulate safe vitamins and minerals as "dangerous drugs" if they exceed 150

41

percent of the so-called recommended daily allowance (RDA) of vitamins and minerals is based on an arbitrary, unscientific, and tainted standard. The RDA standard is established by the Food and Drug Nutrition Board of the National Research Council, which is influenced, dominated and financed in part by the food industry. It represents one of the most scandalous conflicts of interest in the Federal Government.

Since 1968, the RDA list of vitamin needs has changed 65 times. Part of the problem is that there has been no official definition of the word "vitamin." As a result, the board has had no standard for judging what will and what will not be considered a vitamin. Vitamin E, for example, was clinically investigated for almost a quarter of a century before it was grudgingly admitted to the list of essential vitamins.

Vitamin B_{15} (pangamic acid) and vitamin B_{17} (amygdalin and/or similar cyanophoric glucosides) have either been ignored or dismissed in the United States, largely because of the Laetrile (processed vitamin B_{17}) controversy which we will explore in chapter four. But important research has continued in the Soviet Union, which "lifted" the idea from Ernst T. Krebs, Jr., the American biochemist who pioneered the work on vitamin B_{15}. Pangamic acid has been sold *as* vitamin B_{15} in a number of European countries as well as in the United States, even though the FDA and government guidelines do not consider it to be a vitamin.

"SAFE AND EFFECTIVE"

Another problem caused by the FDA is what is euphemistically called the "drug lag." This refers to the time between the development of a new drug or "chemical entity" and the final approval by the FDA to place that product on the market.

When a new drug moves through the Investigational New Drug (IND) procedures of animal testing for "safety and efficacy," it may take anywhere from eight to ten years and can cost up to $20 million in total expenses before it is licensed. Naturally a pharmaceutical company must believe that it will eventually recover these expenses or it will not continue the drug's development. Eli Lilly and Company estimates that the expense it incurs in complying with the regulations of the government in preparing 27,000 forms and reports costs the consumer up to 50 cents per prescription.

The Food, Drug and Cosmetic Act was amended in 1962 as a result of the Thalidomide-tragedy scare. Before that time promoters of drugs had only to prove that those drugs were safe when used in certain specified ways. This requirement was sufficient to ban Thalidomide from use in the United States, and no new regulations were necessary. However, the tragedy that occurred in other countries where the use of Thalidomide was permitted was sufficient to scare some people into giving the FDA more power. Since that time a chemical entity that someone wishes to have licensed as a new drug must be demonstrated in animal tests to be *effective* as well as safe in treating certain conditions.

As a result of the new requirement, the number of new drugs reaching the market has decreased about 60 percent, with only about 15 new drugs being licensed annually now, as compared with approximately 49 licensed annually before 1962. The red tape alone has been one of the key reasons. It has been estimated that up to 200,000 pieces of paperwork must accompany the huge investment in time and money needed to shepherd a new drug from conception to its licensing. Prior to 1962, only about 75 pieces of paper were required.

As the law now stands, only the huge pharmaceutical companies can afford to license new drugs. The smaller companies simply cannot afford the $12 million that is the average cost required. The result is, of course, the elimination of competition in the marketplace and, therefore, fewer drugs available to Americans.

In addition, drugs developed in other countries which could be of help to millions of Americans have been blocked, stymied, or otherwise kept unavailable in this country because of the necessity of proving them effective under the complicated guidelines of the FDA requirements.

The type of person with whom one must deal at the FDA may be seen in the following two examples.

Dr. Theodore Klumpp, former chairman of the Medical Services Task Force of the Hoover Commission, wrote in *The*

Journal of Legal Medicine of a member of the cardiovascular section of the FDA who "boasted that for *nine and one-half years* he blocked the release of any drug for angina pectoris and hypertension on the ground that these were symptoms and not diseases." (Emphasis added.) Of course, all drugs such as aspirin and other pain killers, tranquilizers, and cold remedies have as their purpose to relieve symptoms and not to cure diseases. But then, drugs like aspirin, insulin, and even penicillin would never have been able to pass the current requirements of the FDA for safety and efficacy.

Other FDA officials were described in the following way by Dr. Richard Crout, Director of the Bureau of Drugs of the FDA before the Panel of New Drug Regulation in the Department of Health, Education and Welfare:

> There was absenteeism; there was open drunkenness by several employees, which went on for months; there was intimidation internally; and there was a great deal of what I would call feudalism in bureaucracy.... I can tell you that, in my first year at the FDA—even actually longer than that, 1972, 1973— going to certain kinds of meetings was an extraordinarily peculiar kind of exercise. People—I'm talking about Division directors and their staffs—would engage in a kind of behavior that invited insubordination; people tittered in the corners, throwing spitballs—now I'm describing physicians; people would slouch down in the chair and not respond to questions; and moan-and-groan, the sleeping gestures. This was a kind of behavior I have not seen in any other institution from a grown man.

The result of all of this is, of course, an increased cost to the consumer and taxpayer. Under present laws it costs taxpayers about $1 billion a year to administer the FDA, if you can say it is administered at all. The additional expenses and requirements that the pharmaceutical companies must meet cost the consumer about 50 cents per prescription. Even worse is the cost in human suffering and lives that is brought about by the unavailability of drugs on the American market. It has been estimated that *24 times* the number of Americans who died in Vietnam have died because of the drug lag that exists because of the efficacy clause of the Food, Drug and Cosmetic Act.

In addition, the FDA tries to regulate how the drugs it approves are used and the maximum dosage that can be administered. But the amount of any drug that is needed varies from person to person and from disease to disease, and so what the FDA is really trying to do is to interfere in the relationship between a patient and his chosen physician. Obviously, the physician who is present is a much better judge of what treatment a patient needs than is the FDA.

The idea that there should be some kind of check on the safety (not the efficacy) of drugs is not in itself an evil, alien concept—but the risk of turning to giant government for this information as well as for judgment of effectiveness by bureaucrats who do not practice medicine except from behind a desk should be clear. A large part of the nation's degenerative disease tragedy can be laid directly at the door of giant government in general and the FDA in particular.

MIND POLLUTION—STRESS

Stress is a condition in which the body and its organ systems are placed under strain as a result of the required increase in the functioning of one or more organ systems.

Basically, we recognize physical and emotional stress, but separating them or segmenting them is extremely difficult, if not impossible, in most cases. There are, however, situations in which there is a greater proportion of one over the other. For example, the stress of a pregnancy upon the body of a young woman is mostly physical. However, what woman has ever gone through pregnancy without the emotional fears of whether she will be able to care for the child and whether her husband will continue to love her and care for her and the baby?

Another stress which is primarily physical is undergoing surgery with general anesthetic. In this case there is the accompanying fear of death or of maiming as a result of the surgery, or the fear of being out of control while unconscious. Similarly, when one is suffering from a serious illness due to an infection, there is the fear that something more serious may be wrong, as well as the fear of not being able to function normally because one is not feeling well.

On the other hand, stress that is primarily emotional usually has a definite physical effect. This is often the case

45

when there is a divorce, a separation, a broken love affair, the death of a close member of the family, a boss whom the employee is unable to satisfy, or a job that one is unable to enjoy and in which one feels no sense of accomplishment.

Other examples of emotional stress include dissatisfaction with one's lot in life, boredom and fears of death or of disability. Each and every one of these or any combination of them, or even fears that are locked in the subconscious mind and of which we are unaware on a conscious level, may directly cause or be contributory to diseases that are physically manifested such as ulcers, colitis, heart disease, cancer, colds, and headaches.

Stress is especially prevalent in our hustle-bustle, time-conscious, success-oriented society. And while the effects of stress may vary from person to person, in that some people seem to withstand it better than others, when it is combined with the air, water and food pollution with which we are all bombarded daily, the result is the Killer Disease disaster we are presently enduring.

THE ONSET OF DEGENERATIVE DISEASE

Degenerative diseases are not caused by viruses, bacteria, or parasites, but by the body's inadequate metabolic response to a condition in which the cells of the body are being slowly poisoned by too many of the wrong things or not enough of the right things at the right time.

Arteriosclerotic vascular disease and its allied conditions which are broadly referred to as heart disease, diabetes, cancer, arthritis, emphysema, and probably multiple sclerosis, as well as a number of lesser and, in themselves, nonfatal maladies, are all reflections of this *same* underlying metabolic disorder. Whether it will first appear in an individual as cancer or heart disease or diabetes, or never advance beyond a particularly severe case of hypoglycemia or arthritis, depends upon which tissue has been most insulted by poisonous habits and environment, the extent to which an individual metabolism responds to various stimuli and the extent to which an individual may be more genetically prone to one tissue weakness rather than another.

Although Western medicine is only dimly aware of it, there are indications of the existence of this underlying metabolic disorder. Primarily, these indicators are the silent precursor states of hypoglycemia (low blood sugar) and hypertension (high blood pressure). Millions of Americans are afflicted with one or both of these precursor states, but they may be completely unaware of it. Even though it is now possible to detect hypoglycemia through correct testing procedures and even though hypertension can be discovered with relative ease, most victims of these early warning conditions live from day to day with no knowledge that they have them.

Hypoglycemia, which we will discuss more fully in chapter two, is usually the first hint of trouble. Unfortunately, the great majority of physicians are unable to make an accurate diagnosis of this state—perhaps because of the denial by so many medical people that the state even exists. And even when the state is admitted as existing, orthodox physicians and organizations such as the American Medical Association and the American Diabetes Association deny that most of its accompanying symptoms are, in fact, caused by hypoglycemia. They claim that there is no hard evidence that hypoglycemia causes depression, anxiety, chronic fatigue, allergies, juvenile delinquency, and other behavioral problems such as drug addiction and alcoholism. Of course, when that attitude is taken, the above symptoms are "treated" without understanding their cause, and as a consequence, few patients will be cured. They may be given drugs and tranquilizers or sent from one specialist to another, but when these problems are caused by low blood sugar, they will not disappear until that state is corrected.

More than anything else, degenerative disease begins with problems of carbohydrate metabolism—that is, the sum total of chemical changes and processes involved in the body's handling of the vital organic compounds known as carbohydrates. The initial stage of this problem is hypoglycemia, which generally leads to dysinsulinemia (diabetogenic hypoglycemia), and then to diabetes. It is also often related to obesity, alcoholism, and a large number of emotional disorders ranging from chronic depression to outright schizophrenia. (These

47

mental disorders may also be caused by toxic chemicals and/or deficiencies in specific nutrients.) There is, in addition, a high statistical correlation between diabetes and cancer.

Individual cells are incredibly self-sustaining, self-cleaning, and self-monitoring, but they are also inexorably linked to the rest of the organism and depend upon it for their various needs in relation to their growth and continued existence.

Brain and nerve cells are the most susceptible to nutritional deprivation and/or change. Oxygen and glucose, in that order, are the primary factors which determine whether these cells continue their proper functioning.

Large quantities of refined carbohydrates as well as the continued exposure to toxic chemicals such as lead, mercury, and cadmium affect the division of cells adversely. Tissues can take an enormous amount of abuse or insult, but sooner or later continued insult will lead to aberrant cell division, which is the beginning of degenerative disease.

In addition, the proper functioning of cells depends on a system of enzymes. These are complex catalyzing agents which cause changes in the body. Each enzyme molecule contains one or more of the trace minerals such as magnesium, manganese, copper, zinc, chromium, and potassium, without which the enzyme cannot function properly, causing, in turn, the cells not to function properly. The trace minerals are normally consumed in natural foods, and any deficiency or, on the other side, any overloading of the system with toxic minerals may cause the tissues to break down. It is this type of breakdown that is probably responsible for such degenerative diseases as multiple sclerosis and muscular dystrophy.

When a person is young, leads a relatively healthy life, and moves along at a relatively even keel without enormous amounts of stress, the body may seem to function well. Nevertheless, internal problems may be developing in the form of deposits in his circulatory system and the gradual but insistent insulting of his various organs. An individual may thus function for a long time without being aware of these internal problems. Then one day some kind of stress is put on the system, and suddenly the problems become all too apparent.

The continual ingestion of refined carbohydrates—junk food—practically from birth, and often even before birth because of the eating habits of the mother, helps to create a fatty "bedrock," or matrix, on which heavy toxic minerals may fasten. This action, continued over the years, will cause plaques (deposits) on the walls of arteries. This state is called "hardening of the arteries," or arteriosclerosis.

Hence, denaturalized food consumption is not only an insult to tissues directly, but it also works in conjunction with other elements in our technological society to help further pollute the body. The net result of all this is becoming painfully clear.

Although hardening of the arteries, high blood pressure, and arthritis were once thought to be primarily diseases of the elderly, we now have cases of babies *born* with arthritis, and there is evidence, particularly from the bodies of American soldiers killed during the Korean and Vietnam wars, of significant arteriosclerosis in the majority of the bodies of the soldiers in their early twenties. Cancer, the number two killer in this country, was also formerly thought to be primarily a disease of the aged, but is now striking more and more young people every year.

Diseases of the heart and circulatory system claimed more American lives in 1974 than all other causes of death combined. They killed 1,035,000, which was 54 percent of all deaths that year. Included in that total, heart attacks killed about 665,000, strokes (the end product of high blood pressure and arteriosclerosis) 270,000, rheumatic heart disease 13,300, hypertensive disease 19,000, and congenital heart defects 6,700.

It was estimated in 1974—the last year for which statistics are available—that 30 million Americans had some major form of heart or circulatory disease, and that hypertension, high blood pressure, affected at least 24 million, coronary heart disease another 4 million, rheumatic heart disease 1,800,000, and stroke 1,810,000.

What does all of this cost? While a total figure that includes all of the indirect or hidden costs for heart disease is difficult to come by, the cost has been estimated to be *at least* $27 billion per year. Included in this figure are the nearly $3 billion simply to pay physicians and nurses, $7 billion for hospitals and nursing homes, $700 million or more for heart medication, $1.1 billion to build the large hospital research and surgical facilities, and a known $8.6 billion in lost wages.

Trailing not far behind and rapidly gaining on heart disease is the world's second major killer, cancer. Both the number of cases and the fatalities have reached all-time highs with about 400,000 deaths a year in the United States from cancer or its orthodox treatments and complications and 675,000 new cases of cancer diagnosed every year. It is the only "natural" cause of death that showed a big increase in America between 1973 and 1975. Cancer now kills about 1,100 Americans *daily*.

Because of its elusiveness, its ability to kill quickly or cause long, drawn-out bouts of suffering, and the lack of success in curbing it, cancer has developed a kind of mystique in which the average person immediately associates it with death.

Total spending on health care in the United States was $140 billion in 1976, with national health insurance plans and programs expected to raise that figure well beyond $200 billion within five years. About 80 percent of this is spent on the treatment of degenerative diseases in all their phases. Thus, only a small amount of the nation's total health-care monies is spent on the infectious diseases, parasites, and deficiencies that at one time were the major killers of the Western world.

Today, those diseases that are the result of the body's breakdown in metabolism—the Killer Diseases—are filling the hospitals and clinics and fattening the pockets of those in the health-care delivery industry, which would be more appropriately called "the sick business." The $150 to $300 a day hospital rooms, skyrocketing medical insurance costs, enormous medical fees and salaries, the ever more expensive drugs pushed by the pharmaceutical cartel, and an ever expanding armamentarium of expensive gadgetry of all kinds designed to provide the latest diagnostic techniques for a civilization that is getting sicker and sicker are all parts of this business.

It is a gravy train—for the developer and pusher of expensive drugs, the network of drug distributors, the clinics and hospitals and their builders and planners, the manufacturers and distributors of the awesomely expensive and complicated medical machinery, the medical specialists and paramedical teams, the surgeons, the anesthesiologists, and the dispensers, recipients, and handlers of billions of dollars in public and private research money.

CRISIS CARE VERSUS
THE NEW BREED

American medicine has become, more than anything else, "crisis" medicine. A person is not treated, or even encouraged to see a physician, until there is some symptom of a malfunction within his body. And it is the symptom, *not the cause* of that symptom, that is most often treated. This type of "health care," called allopathy, is the one practiced almost exclusively in this country. Its direct result is "specialized" and "fragmented" medicine in which everyone has his own set of a small number of symptoms at which he is an "expert" at blocking and checking and which sends the suffering patient from, for example, the dermatologist to the internist to the psychiatrist to the surgeon while each tries to find a "cure" for some one or two of his symptoms.

In the case of hypoglycemia alone, the sufferer may present such a myriad of symptoms that his treatment may well seem to fall within a dozen medical specialties and he may go from one walnut paneled office to another, gulp down a dozen medications and drugs, or undergo guinea pig testing of some new drugs before a physician correctly diagnoses his disease state as that of glucose metabolism dysfunction—the body's inability to maintain adequate or normal blood sugar levels in the bloodstream—if, indeed, he is lucky enough to find a physician who is able to make this determination.

Allopathic, fragmented crisis medicine naturally leads to the exaltation of surgery as the *creme de la creme* of modern medicine. The best-paid and most respected individual on the medical team is the one who can cut, bypass or lop off better than his fellow practitioners. A recent congressional committee report indicated that in the United States alone some 2.4 million surgeries costing $4 billion in 1974 and taking 12,000 lives were found to be unnecessary. They were done because that is "medicine as usual."

The American Medical Association, virtually a closed union shop, is almost entirely in the hands of the allopathic, medical-specialist school. To break step with fragmented crisis medicine is to do so without the blessings of the AMA and to

51

risk the wrath of "peer review"—usually in the form of state or local boards of medical examiners and licensers—a practice that subverts the very meaning of the Hippocratic Oath.

The advent of allopathy as "Establishment" medicine is understandable because of its success in dealing with infections, the major health problem at one time. It is also understandable that the drug producers should want this type of medicine to continue to dominate the field. These two Siamese twins of modern health care dominate advertising, propaganda, and information, control and publish the majority of medical texts and health journals, and manipulate the raising and spending of vast sums of "research" money.

It has gotten so bad that allopathic medicine itself in many instances is a cure *worse* than the disease, and it is involved to a considerable degree in the rapid rise of the iatrogenic, or "doctor-caused," illnesses and fatalities.

In spite of the maze of tests and paperwork required by the FDA, some drugs seem to be rushed on the market, somehow circumventing the red tape, while others wait for years and years without added impetus for development. Thus many drugs are unleashed on the market that have serious toxic effects on people in spite of the fact that all drugs are supposedly checked for "safety and efficacy" in animals—as if tests on animals can really tell what effect the drugs will have on humans. As a result, many drugs are used on patients in what amount to guinea pig experiments.

The result is that the number of patients who die from drug side-effects in the United States is between 6,000 and 12,000 annually. About 18 percent of patients already hospitalized suffer from adverse reactions from drugs. It is also estimated that for every drug prescription filled in the United States a dollar must be spent on dealing with complications which arise from using the drug. Five percent of the patients hospitalized in the United States are there because of the effects of drugs they are taking, not because they have any disease.

Dr. Edgar Berman, the personal physician of Senator Hubert Humphrey and the author of *The Solid Gold Stethoscope,* is among the physicians who have spoken out against medicine as usual. In a blistering indictment of the abuses of his profession, Dr. Berman was quoted as saying that "some 14,000 to 16,000 persons die each year because of the two to three million unnecessary operations performed." He estimates that hospitals actually produce 5 million new cases of disease a year and that 1.4 million hospitalizations are caused by prescribed drugs. He reprimanded those doctors who "shuffle patients through their offices like cattle" and claimed that far too many physicians are more interested in money than in human lives.

Any dissent from the established line of medicine as usual, any rattling of the allopathic cage, is sure to bring serious attacks on the dissenters—as chiropractors, homeopaths, and naturopaths can attest. But that is not new. Entrenched establishments have throughout history made short shrift of dissenters and disturbers. As a result, in science in general and medicine in particular, virtually every major breakthrough has been brought about by individuals or groups who, operating outside the mainstream of American medicine, ran the risk of being classified as charlatans or quacks before "orthodoxy" finally accepted their ideas.

And, today, not all physicians and practitioners of the medical arts are in agreement with the practice of allopathy. With the brutal and gruesome statistics of degenerative disease before them and the obvious failure of medicine as usual to deal with these Killer Diseases, the dissenters are beginning to speak out forcefully against Establishment medicine. A new breed of young—and not always so young—Turks have arisen to do battle with the entrenched forces of the allopathic American Medical Association and its friends, the drug companies and food processors.

These dissenting physicians see the tragedy of degenerative disease and, indeed, disease in general, in quite a different way than does the Establishment.

To begin with, they believe that the path to good health lies in prevention far more than treatment, and this attitude alone places them one cosmos removed from the health-care delivery industry. Who ever heard of a *prevention* center? The money is not in prevention but in treatment—because under the status quo it is a certainty that virtually every American will have to spend an increasingly large chunk of his life, be it in his "senior" years or much sooner, in clinics and hospitals. Prevention is simply not a part of the average medical mentality or usual medical education in this country.

Secondly, the young Turks believe that if treatment is necessary, it must be based on the whole man. No disease or condition exists by itself. It must be conceived of as linked to everything else in the body, and the body must be conceived of as linked to the mind. Thus these doctors regard degenerative diseases as systemic, chronic metabolic disorders, not a gaggle of separate, fragmented diseases to be dealt with by separate specialists in fragmented medicine.

They argue that "treatment" of degenerative diseases should first and foremost be the prevention of these states. But, faced with the reality that the vast majority of the patients they see are suffering from one or more degenerative disease conditions, they believe that the answer, if an answer is still available and degeneration has not progressed to the point of no return, is in the restoration of the metabolic balance of the body. This is accomplished through vitamins, minerals, enzymes, a complete change in eating habits, adequate physical exercise, and a change in the stressful attitudes of life.

Most of these physicians would agree that allopathic approaches to medicine have done a commendable job in the treatment of specific infections and sometimes in the treatment of degenerative disease. They would not agree, however, that allopathic approaches are *always* appropriate. They point out that this preoccupation of the medical community with causes of diseases becomes an erroneous goal in the case of degenerative diseases. In these cases it is often not the case that they are caused by something, but by the *lack* of something. Thus, the researchers' hunt for the human, cancer-causing virus becomes a misdirected quest—just as bypass surgery is frequently an unnecessary and useless tool in the treatment of heart disease.

Since the emphasis of these dissenting physicians is on prevention as opposed to treatment, they pose a monumental threat to the vested interest groups in the sick business. And since, even in treatment, they rely on nutritional change and natural foods as the primary metabolic weapons, they also pose a challenge to food processors and the producers and distributors of expensive and frequently toxic drugs.

There is no single description for the approach these doctors are following in medicine. Perhaps the best phrases are "metabolic" or "holistic" medicine, but they may call themselves many different things. Primarily they are involved in prevention, nutrition, metabolic therapy, and megavitamin therapy

—the latter frequently falling under the unwieldy label of "orthomolecular therapy." They may also be involved in other effective but unorthodox treatments such as chelation for cardiovascular disease. But whatever they call themselves, what they are doing is nothing short of revolutionary: they are practicing medicine based on the belief that man must be viewed holistically, that there is a need for the proper balance of all the ingredients within man's metabolism and a balance in his relationship to the environment. They are *returning* to the original concepts of ancient health care, which stressed natural prevention rather than treatment.

They are also beginning to fulfill the prophecy of Thomas Edison: "The doctor of the future will give no medicine but will interest his patients in the care of the human frame, in diet, and in the cause and prevention of disease."

A number of organizations have been formed for the purpose of distributing educational information to physicians and paramedical personnel and to participate in research and development of holistic, metabolic, and preventive medicine. These groups include the American Academy of Medical Preventics, whose members have been pioneers in the fight for the recognition of chelation therapy in the treatment of heart disease, the International Academy of Preventive Medicine, the Academy of Orthomolecular Psychiatry, the International College of Applied Nutrition, and the International Academy of Metabology.

In addition, there are organizations such as the National Health Federation, which has long championed preventive medicine and nutritional therapy, the Committee for Freedom of Choice in Cancer Therapy, Inc., which brings together people interested in the holistic approach to the prevention and management of cancer, and the Association for Chelation Therapy (ACT). The latter three groups are organizations that are oriented toward the dissemination of educational material to the lay public as well as to any medical person who is interested. The addresses of all of these nonprofit organizations are provided in appendix D for anyone who is interested in more information.

The task of these doctors is formidable. Civilized man *is* polluting himself to death. We run absolutely no risk of increased "population explosion" since, if degenerative disease continues to kill, maim and cripple on the scale it has already reached, the Western world will lose a major portion of its population in a relatively short period of time.

Crisis medicine, fragmented medicine, specialty medicine is not solving the problem—it is actually making it worse. What we must have is a complete reform not only of medicine but also of the nutritional habits of the civilized world. The alternative is the self-destruction of man.

TWO

In the Beginning, Sugar

GLUCOSE METABOLISM DYSFUNCTION

We have indicated that low blood sugar—hypoglycemia—is the precursor state or "early warning system" for a whole host of interlocking degenerative diseases. The disease is rarely diagnosed until it is well on its way to becoming something more serious, but the symptoms should not be ignored for they are frequently the early warning signs of eventual diabetes, arthritis, arteriosclerosis, and even cancer.

In this book we have grouped the sequential disease states, of which hypoglycemia is merely step one, under the single umbrella term *glucose metabolism dysfunction* (GMD). GMD is a state brought about by the abnormal function of one or more of the five different organ systems responsible for glucose homeostasis—that is, the optimum function of blood sugar. The five systems involved are the hypothalamus, the pituitary, the pancreas, the adrenals, and the liver. Hypoglycemia, dysinsulinemia, and diabetes are, therefore, different stages of the same disease state that are differentiated by the different type of malfunction involved. This is similar to a situation in which a person might have acute tonsillitis, chronic tonsillitis, follicular tonsillitis, or exudative tonsillitis; these are all forms of tonsillitis that are differentiated on the basis of the different type of infection and the appearance of the tonsils.

Glucose metabolism dysfunction may be manifested in any one of a number of ways: hypoglycemia, glucose intolerance, dysinsulinemia (diabetogenic hypoglycemia), and diabetes. Alcoholism and even schizophrenia may result from GMD.

GMD, per se, is rarely ever diagnosed, due to the unusual absence of physical findings that the physician can correlate. There is practically nothing in GMD that a physician can send off to a laboratory for examination, no composite of clinical evidence that can be gathered to make a diagnosis based on physical findings. The complaints of the GMD-suffering patient sound like so many other things that the examining doctor may conclude that some other specialist should be seen, or, more frequently, that the only thing needed for the depression, nervousness, or fatigue is a tranquilizer or stimulant.

In the majority of GMD cases, physicians do not bother to listen to or become interested in the patient's *total history*. It simply takes too much time and may cut into a busy practice in which patients are practically stacked up in the waiting room to see the man with the stethoscope. Failure to take into account the patient's total history and failure to correlate the sum total of these complaints with GMD and administer a proper six-hour glucose tolerance test, as well as orthodoxy's ambivalent views about hypoglycemia, are the reasons why GMD is the most misdiagnosed or simply "missed" malady in the medical world today.

The importance of discovering and treating hypoglycemia can be seen in the following statistic: 80 percent of untreated hypoglycemics as opposed to only 20 percent of treated hypoglycemics will eventually end up as diabetics. In addition, a significant number of diabetics also develop cancer. And by the time arteriosclerosis is diagnosed, the "sugar junkie" is apt to be well on the way to death from heart disease.

Yet, as essential as it is to detect and treat hypoglycemia, American medical orthodoxy, during most of this century, has tended to deny that the situation even exists and has argued that refined sugar and refined carbohydrates do *not* really hurt us. The American Medical Association and the American Diabetes Association have stated in publications that there is no symptom caused by eating sugar, or even from having low blood sugar, and that there is no good evidence that hypoglycemia causes behavioral problems in children, depression, chronic fatigue, allergies, or even drug addiction and alcoholism.

But in a study done a few years ago in New York in which 100 skid row alcoholics were given six-hour glucose tolerance tests, it was found that every single one of them had some form of glucose metabolism dysfunction—that is, either hypoglycemia, diabetes, or dysinsulinemia, which is the middle stage between hypoglycemia and diabetes.

As to whether the blood sugar problem carries with it a behavioral ramification, we need only examine the study made on the Qolla Indians of Bolivia and Peru. Described as the meanest and cruelest people who have ever lived, they have been studied carefully, and their chronicled history covers more than 350 years.

One study was made by a Californian who gave glucose tolerance tests to 66 male Qollas. Their traditional diet is atrocious, consisting primarily of refined carbohydrates. The murder rate for the village studied was 55 per 100,000 per year—which is a great deal higher than the figures for the United States, which most people consider frighteningly violent. In fact, if the United States had the same murder rate as the Qollas, there would be 115,000 murders here per year.

Hypoglycemia was diagnosed in the majority of the Qollas tested. However, the most interesting thing discovered in the study was that the most aggressive men in the community were those who had the least severe cases of hypoglycemia. Those who had the most severe hypoglycemia were the least aggressive and committed the fewest murders—simply because they did not have the energy to fight.

There is an automatic mechanism in man that regulates the level of glucose in the body. When sugar or caffeine is ingested, the glucose level is raised and the pancreas is stimulated, causing the release of insulin, a hormone which is essential for carbohydrate metabolism. The insulin forces the glucose level down through two mechanisms: (1) it causes the liver to convert glucose into the storage form of sugar, glycogen, which cannot be used by the individual cells of the body in that form, and (2) it causes the transfer of glucose across cellular membranes. When the glucose level drops to the "fasting level," which is the lowest optimum level where the body can still function normally, the adrenal gland is stimulated and releases adrenalin, which in turn causes the blood sugar level to rise as the liver converts the glycogen back to glucose.

But when a person has hypoglycemia, this automatic mechanism does not function properly as a result of the overstimulation of the pancreas by the excessive amounts of refined carbohydrates and caffeine that have been ingested. In this state, the pancreas releases an excessive amount of insulin, and this causes the glucose level to plunge below the fasting level. Then the adrenal gland must work overtime trying to raise the blood sugar level again. The continual overload of the system causes adrenal exhaustion.

By this point the hypoglycemic has multiple symptoms of everything from nervousness, irritability, and exhaustion to antisocial behavior, leg cramps, crying spells, indecisiveness, twitching and jerking of the muscles, and even suicidal tendencies.

Dr. Stephen Gyland, himself a hypoglycemic, did much to bring the attention of American medicine to bear on the long ignored problem of low blood sugar. He endured an agonizing odyssey in which he was examined by 14 specialists and at three major clinics. Dr. Gyland was diagnosed at one major clinic as having a brain tumor, at another as having diabetes, and was finally told that he had a psychiatric disorder that would necessitate his retirement from medical practice because he was no longer capable of practicing medicine.

The observations of his newly graduated M.D. son led to a six-hour glucose tolerance test and his problem was finally diagnosed correctly and ultimately cured through diet.

In the course of trying to control his own illness Dr. Gyland came across the original paper published on the subject by Seale Harris, M.D., in a 1924 *Journal of the American Medical Association*. Harris studied and categorized the symptoms of 600 hypoglycemia patients, and he established the following list of symptoms. Beside each symptom is given the percentage of hypoglycemic patients in which it occurred.

Nervousness .... 94 %
Irritability .... 89 %
Exhaustion .... 87 %
Faintness, dizziness, tremor, cold sweats, and/or
    weak spells .... 86 %
Depression .... 77 %
Vertigo, dizziness .... 73 %
Drowsiness .... 72 %
Headaches .... 71 %

Digestive disturbances .... 69 %
Forgetfulness .... 67 %
Insomnia ....:................. 62 %
Constant worrying, unprovoked anxieties ...... 62 %
Mental confusion .... 57 %
Internal trembling .... 57 %
Palpitation of heart and/or rapid pulse .... 54 %
Muscle pains .... 53 %
Numbness .... 51 %
Indecisiveness .... 50 %
Unsocial, asocial or antisocial behavior .... 47 %
Crying spells .... 46 %
Lack of sex drive in females .... 44 %
Allergies .... 43 %
Incoordination .... 43 %
Leg cramps .... 43 %
Lack of concentration .... 42 %
Blurred vision .... 40 %
Twitching and jerking of muscles .... 40 %
Itching and crawling sensations of the skin .... 39 %
Gasping for breath .... 37 %
Smothering spells .... 34 %
Staggering .... 34 %
Sighing and yawning .... 30 %
Impotence in males .... 29 %
Unconsciousness .... 27 %
Night terrors, nightmares .... 27 %
Rheumatoid arthritis .... 24 %
Phobias, fears .... 23 %
Neurodermatitis .... 21 %
Suicidal intent .... 20 %
Nervous breakdown .... 17 %
Convulsions .... 2 %

In a paper read before a local medical organization associated with the American Medical Association, Dr. Gyland reported that among the many mistaken diagnoses that were
made on these patients were Meniere's syndrome (dizziness,
loss of hearing, and noises in the ears), cerebral arteriosclerosis, chronic bronchial asthma, senile palsy (Parkinson's syndrome), menopause, alcoholism, and diabetes. There was one
correct diagnosis of hyperinsulinism (low blood sugar), but
treatment had been based on the consumption of candy bars!

Harper Health Indicator Test

0	1	2	3	
				Tired all the time
				Hungry between meals or at night
				Depressed
				Insomnia
				Wake up after a few hours' sleep
				Fearful (overwhelmed by people, places, or things)
				Can't decide easily
				Can't concentrate
				Poor memory
				Worry frequently
				Feel insecure or low self-image
				Highly emotional
				Moody
				Cry easily, or feel like crying inside
				Fits of anger
				Magnify insignificant details (make mountains out of molehills)
				Eat candy, cake, cookies, or drink soda pop
				Eat bread, pasta, potatoes, rice, or beans
				Consume alcohol
				Drink more than 3 cups of coffee or cola drinks daily
				Crave candy, soda, or coffee between meals or mid-afternoon
				Can't work well under pressure
				Headaches
				Sleepy during the day
				Sleepy or drowsy after meals
				Lack of energy
				Reduced initiative
				Can't get started in the morning
				Eat when nervous
				Stomach cramps or "nervous stomach"
				Allergies: asthma, hay fever, skin rash, sinus trouble, etc.
				Fatigue relieved by eating
				Suicidal thoughts or tendencies, feelings of hopelessness
				Bored
				Bad dreams
				Irritable before meals
				Heart beats fast (palpitations)
				Get shaky inside if hungry
				Feel faint if meal is delayed
				Ulcers, gastritis, chronic indigestion, abdominal bloating
				Cold hands or feet
				Trembling (shaking) of the hands
				Blurred vision
				Bleeding gums

				Dizziness, giddiness, or light-headedness
				Aware of breathing heavily
				Bruise easily
				Reduced sex drive
				Uncoordination (drop or bump into things)
				Sweating excessively
				Unsocial or antisocial behavior
				Muscle twitching or cramps
				Skin aches
				Phobias
				Hallucinations
				Convulsions
0				TOTALS (number of checks in column times column number)

TOTAL OF COLUMNS 1, 2, & 3:

The American Medical Association never saw fit to print Dr. Gyland's article in any of its journals, but it was printed in a Brazilian medical journal. Thus, anyone interested in Gyland's work may read the article—if he understands Portuguese.

This is only one example of the continuing blindness of American medicine when it comes to recognizing glucose metabolism dysfunction.

The best way to find out if a person has hypoglycemia is to administer a six-hour glucose tolerance test, which measures blood sugar and reveals the body's ability or inability to metabolize refined carbohydrates. But before worrying about a glucose tolerance test, a person can learn whether there is a probable need for such a test by taking the Harper Health Indicator Test on pages 62–63.

Check off each symptom that you have according to its severity. A *0* in the column indicates you never have the symptom, *1* means that it is mild when it occurs and/or only occurs occasionally, *2* means that it is moderate and/or occurs at least once a week, and *3* means that it is severe and occurs frequently.

Add up the number of checks in a single column and multiply that number by the number at the head of that column. Thus, if you have 10 checks in the column headed by 3, multiply 10 times 3 and the total for that column is 30. Repeat this process for the other columns and then add columns 1, 2, and 3 together. From the total of the three columns you can ascertain the probability of whether or not you have a glucose metabolism problem without taking the six-hour test.

Of course, the fact that a person has any of the symptoms listed need not mean that he has low blood sugar. Obviously, almost everyone has had every one of the symptoms at some time or another. The suspicion that they may be attributable to low blood sugar springs from the number and frequency of a combination of these symptoms.

If you have done the test accurately and added the results correctly, and scored 15 or less, you have only a 2 percent probability of having an abnormal glucose tolerance test. If your score falls between 15 and 20, the probability is raised to 5 percent. If the score is between 20 and 25 the probability goes up to 50 percent, and between 25 and 35 it is 75 percent. If the score is between 35 and 45 the probability of glucose metabolism dysfunction is 90 percent. Anything in excess of 45 points indicates a 98 percent likelihood of an abnormal glucose tolerance test.

Run properly, the glucose tolerance test involves taking a fasting blood sugar reading and then giving the patient 100 grams of sugar in a noncola-flavored beverage. (Unfortunately, at the present time, one of the most common beverages given in the test is Glucola. This drink is cola-flavored and like all colas contains caffeine. Thus, the use of Glucola in the test to serve as a "challenge" to the body has a completely undesirable effect because the caffeine causes an abnormal secretion of adrenalin and may invalidate the results of the test by causing a "false normal" reading.)

After the beverage has been consumed a reading of the blood sugar level is taken at least every half hour. This can be done by withdrawing a drop or two of blood from the finger. If a device such as the Ames Reflectance Meter is used, an accurate reading can be obtained within 90 seconds. This technique is obviously superior to those in which blood is withdrawn from the arm and sent to a laboratory for processing, with the results being returned at some time in the future long after the patient has completed the test. When a reading is immediately available, the physician can follow what is happening in the body from moment to moment and thus can know exactly when additional blood sugar readings should be taken and have them performed then. Notice, for example, in figure 14 (page 73) that if readings were taken only at prearranged half-hour intervals, the drop in blood sugar to 45 would not have been seen. In some cases, being unaware of such drops in glucose levels can lead to an incorrect diagnosis.

If a person metabolizes glucose adequately, the result of the glucose tolerance test will be "normal." In these tests, the morning fasting blood sugar will be between 80 and 100 milligrams percent. The patient then drinks the beverage containing the 100 grams of sugar. The one-hour level should show an elevation of blood sugar of between 50 and 100 percent above fasting blood sugar level. Thus, for example, if the fasting level is 90 milligrams, the one-hour level should be between 135 and 180 milligrams. Two hours after the ingestion of the "glucose challenge"—that is, the sugar-bearing drink—the blood sugar should have dropped back down to within 10 percent of the fasting level and remain in that range for the remainder of the six-hour test. Thus, to continue with the example of someone whose fasting blood sugar is 90, the two-hour level should be between 81 and 99 milligrams and it should vary in that range for the remainder of the six hours.

An example of someone with a normal glucose tolerance test can be seen in figure 9. The figures at the top of the graph indicate the time in hours, and the light lines in between these figures indicate half-hour intervals. The glucose level is indicated on the left side of the chart in milligram percent. The gray area represents the normal range in blood sugar levels. The woman whose test results are shown complained of being hungry, nervous, and irritable and of having hot flashes—symptoms similar to those in people who have hypoglycemia. But in this case the test shows that their cause must be found elsewhere; they are not the result of glucose metabolism dysfunction.

Deviation from the pattern described above as normal in glucose tolerance tests reflects some form of glucose metabolism dysfunction.

In figure 10 we see the typical curve of a hypoglycemic. The test is that of a 34-year-old woman whose primary complaints were of shakiness, dizziness, light-headedness, and excessive hunger. She starts with a fasting blood sugar level of about 110, it elevates to 180 milligrams within 30 minutes and then drops back within an hour to 144. At that point her adrenal gland is stimulated, and the adrenalin it releases sends the blood sugar back up to 160. Then the enormous amount of insulin secreted by the pancreas depresses the blood sugar

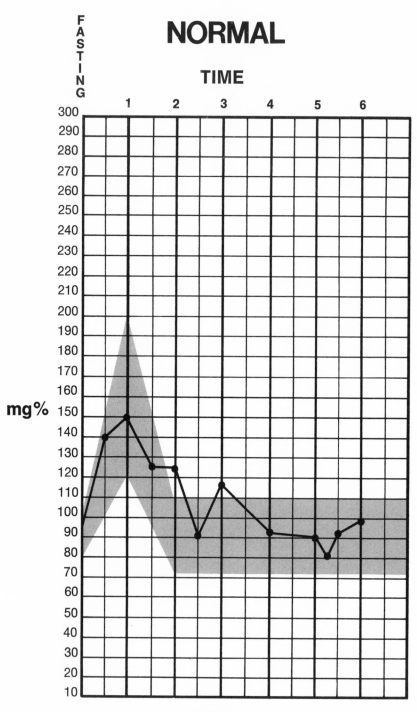

FIGURE 9

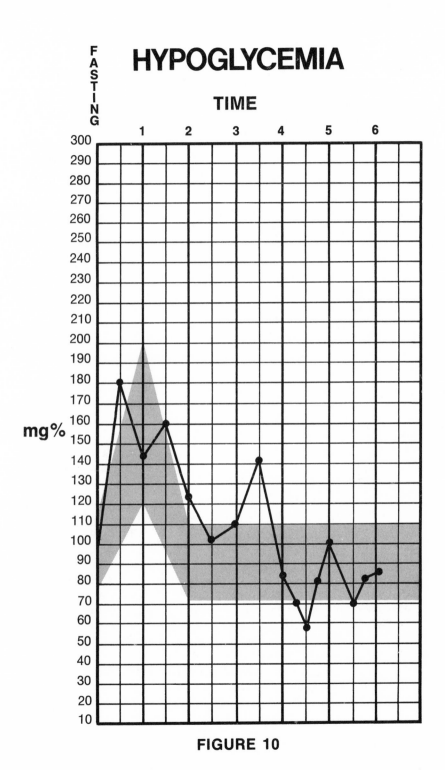

FIGURE 10

again until it reaches 100. At this point there is another adrenal response, which forces the blood sugar up to 144 again, at which point the insulin once more depresses it back down, falling all the way to 52 this time. This is a typical example of the roller-coaster effect of the pancreatic and adrenal functions in a hypoglycemic.

Figure 11 shows the result of a glucose tolerance test taken by a 40-year-old man. He complained of nervousness, shakiness, and severe hunger. Notice that at one point there is a drop to 22 milligrams. According to textbooks, people begin to pass out below the level of 50 and death occurs at the level of 25 or below. Obviously the textbooks are not always correct. Even so, this man does have an extremely severe case of hypoglycemia. His body has learned to compensate for this drop in blood sugar through the adrenal response, but it is this response that makes him shaky and nervous. The adrenalin causes a rise in blood pressure, pulse rate, and muscle tension and forces blood from the skin surfaces into the muscles. This is the so-called fight-or-flight mechanism that helps a person in danger either defend himself or escape. It also causes a rise in blood sugar.

Hypoglycemia follows many patterns, and the test results show many different curves, but the symptoms remain the same. Organizations such as the American Medical Association and the American Diabetic Association like to play the numbers game: "hypoglycemia occurs only when the blood sugar level drops to 50 milligrams or below." Otherwise, they say, it should not be called hypoglycemia. But numbers mean nothing to the cells of the body. When the cells no longer have the ability to perform normally due to nutritional deficiencies, the body malfunctions and causes the symptoms of hypoglycemia—and this is the case whether the blood sugar level drops to 45 or drops only to 55 milligrams percent.

If all hypoglycemics are left untreated—that is, if they go without a therapy program of nutrients, vitamins, and minerals—as many as 80 percent will end up as diabetics eventually. Persons with a heredity pattern of diabetes may develop that condition even if they are treated as hypoglycemics. However, most treated hypoglycemics can assume that they have stopped the sugar disease toboggan if they follow an adequate therapy program.

The test results of a typical early diabetic are seen in figure

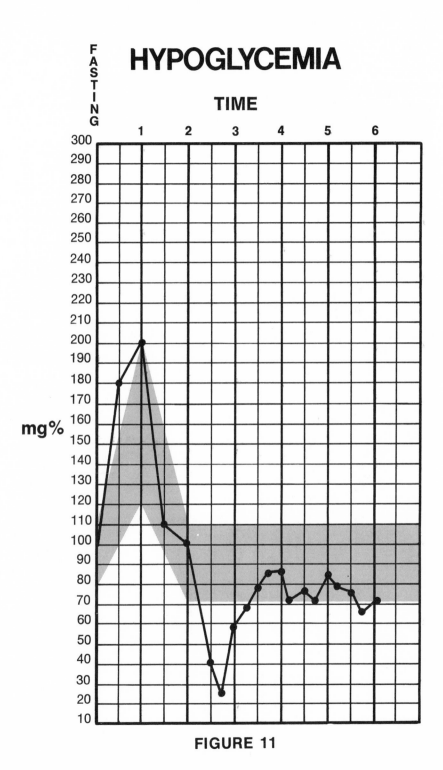

FIGURE 11

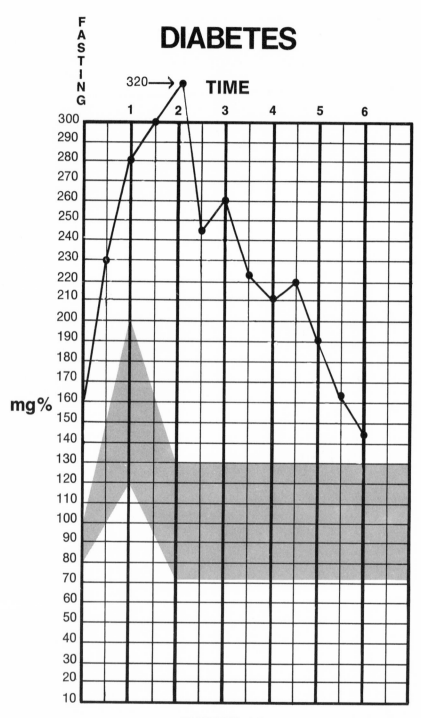

FIGURE 12

12. His fasting blood sugar is 160; it elevates to 320, then gradually drops back, but never goes below 144. This man has some of the same symptoms that hypoglycemics exhibit, but other of his symptoms are worse; they include shakiness, blurred vision, depression, and difficulty in breathing. All these disturbances reflect a malfunction in the systems of the body that handle glucose metabolism. Diabetics frequently have other diseases concurrently with diabetes since it is a multisystem disease.

Dysinsulinemia (diabetogenic hypoglycemia) is the intermediate stage between hypoglycemia and diabetes. In figure 13 we see the test results of a typical dysinsulinemic. There is a severe elevation of the blood sugar in the first two hours, and it does not return to the normal limit by the end of that time. Then there is an adrenal response that sends the blood sugar back up to 220, followed this time by a catastrophic drop to 42.

Under most of the current methods of testing glucose tolerance, the entire test does not extend beyond two or three hours. If this were the type of test administered here, the doctor would notice the fluctuations from 115 to 190 to 450 after an hour and a half and then to 132 at the two-hour level, and he would undoubtedly be puzzled. Most doctors would probably conclude that this individual was diabetic and place him on insulin or an insulin-producing drug, which would make his condition worse, not better. However, by testing the patient for six hours rather than only three, a physician would have all the information needed to make an accurate diagnosis.

In fact, insulin cannot be said to be the cure for diabetes, even when properly diagnosed. Before the use of insulin in Great Britain, deaths from diabetes were 112 per million in 1925. After its introduction in 1926, deaths from diabetes rose to 115 per million, and the rate has continued to rise: there were approximately 174 diabetes deaths per million in the United States in 1974. These figures certainly show that insulin alone is not the way to cure or even control diabetes. The way to prevent diabetes is to cut down or eliminate sugar consumption, and this fact was recognized by the discoverer of insulin, Dr. Frederick Banting, who said: "In the United States the incidence of diabetes has increased proportionately with the per capita consumption of sugar."

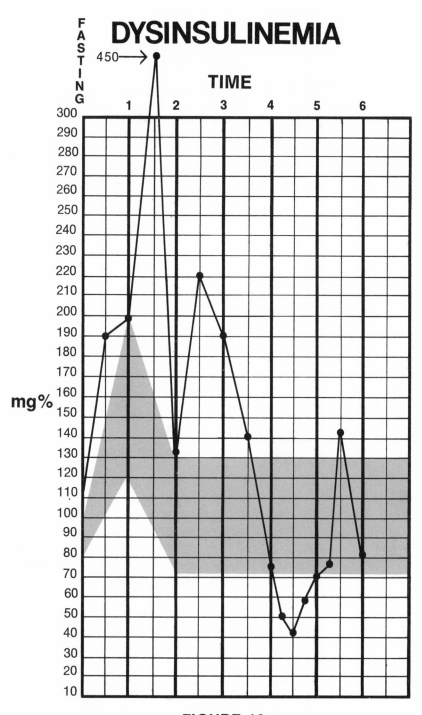

FIGURE 13

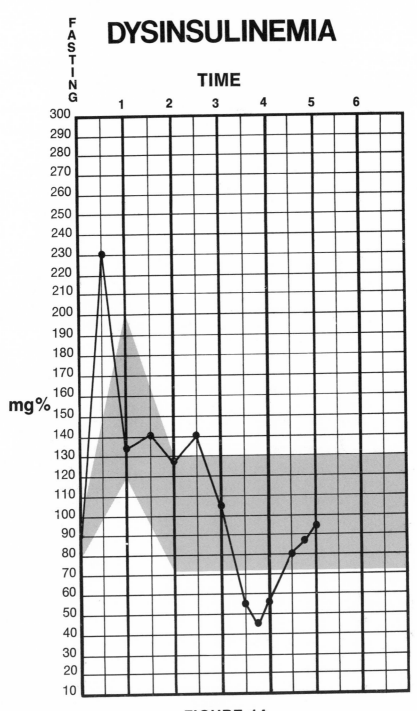

FIGURE 14

In figure 14 we see the test results of a woman with dysinsulinemia. There was an elevation at the two-hour period, with a severe drop to 42. At that point she had hot flashes, a headache, and shakiness, became argumentative, and exaggerated minor difficulties.

If all of this sounds familiar, it should. These symptoms describe the state of a large portion of our population. The American housewife is particularly susceptible because of the stress caused by her boredom and dissatisfaction with life. After a long day alone or with small children, doing chores that require little or no mental effort, her husband comes home from work, gives her a peck on the cheek, and collapses in front of the television set to watch anything and everything, but he pays little attention to her or the children.

She begins the day with several cups of coffee and possibly a cigarette or two instead of breakfast and thus continues her destructive cycle. In fact, the sugar and caffeine are not the only things here related to blood sugar problems. British researchers have found that relatively heavy smoking creates a desire for more caffeine and sugar.

The buying habits of the American housewife are often the key to glucose metabolism problems in her family. Influenced by the incessant stream of televised and printed propaganda as well as the habits she may have inherited from her own mother, the foods she buys and prepares for her family are often those that are major contributors to the glucose metabolism calamity of the Western world.

But when the wife is under treatment for blood sugar problems, it is the husband who often turns out to be the biggest obstacle to the management of the condition. He often feels threatened either consciously or subconsciously by his wife's favorable response to therapy. This is particularly true when the wife, through rigid adherence to her eating program, feels better, has more energy, and becomes thinner and more attractive. As a result, he often makes an effort to sabotage her program by eating foods she is not allowed to have or by otherwise tempting her to slip back into her old habits.

To the greatest extent possible, the eating program (see below) should be a family affair, with the patient adhering rigidly to the plan and the remainder of the family adhering to it in a less rigid manner. This is the best preventive measure anyone can take against degenerative diseases.

As we have indicated, glucose metabolism dysfunction is usually a gradually developing disease in which the individual goes from normal to hypoglycemic to dysinsulinemic to diabetic if left untreated. There is, however, one exception to this progression, and that is the juvenile diabetic in whom these steps are bypassed. In such cases, apparently as a result of a hereditary predisposition to diabetes, a young person may jump from having a normal glucose metabolism to being diabetic.

In the majority of people, however, the onset of diabetes when they are adults results from environmental rather than hereditary factors. It is caused by untreated blood sugar problems and the rapidity of the progression depends here, as in the onset of other types of glucose metabolism dysfunction, on which tissues have been most severely damaged by environmental pollution and emotional and physical stresses, including the stress of food pollution upon the body.

THE HARPER EATING PLAN FOR GMD

Four things are necessary to reverse glucose metabolism dysfunction problems.

(1) Eating only the proper types of food.

(2) Eating at the proper time intervals as determined by the six-hour glucose tolerance test, or every two to three hours when proper testing is unavailable.

(3) Adding specific vitamins and minerals to the diet. These are the raw materials for the building of base products in carbohydrate metabolism—gluco-corticoids and adrenalin by the adrenal gland, insulin by the pancreas, and proper liver function for conversion of glucose to glycogen and glycogen to glucose.

(4) Where appropriate, reducing one's weight to normal and maintaining that weight. This is essential because a reduction in weight increases the concentration of enzymes and hormones for the body's chemical reactions.

When these steps are followed, 85 percent of patients will respond within six to twelve months. Of the patients who respond, 50 percent will show a marked improvement within three days. The other 50 percent will feel worse during the first week of the program, about the same as before beginning the program in the second week and will only begin to show improvement at the end of three weeks.

The 15 percent who will not improve using only these four steps require specific antihypoglycemic and antihyperglycemic agents such as Dilantin, Belladonna, antispasmodic agents, digestive enzymes or aids, and/or adrenal cortical extracts (ACE).

The proper diet for correction of low blood sugar includes proteins, vegetables, and fruits. All refined carbohydrates and caffeine are eliminated from the diet and overweight persons should also eliminate most fats. The complete diet can be found in appendix A.

In the beginning, each feeding should include (1) a small piece of fruit or vegetable plus (2) either one ounce of unprocessed cheese; two ounces of red meat, poultry (without the skin) or seafood; three ounces of low-fat cottage cheese; or one cup of unflavored yogurt.

Moderate amounts of red meat are allowed as excellent sources of protein, but for other health reasons, including the prevention of heart disease and cancer, it is recommended that other sources of protein be used as well. The average American consumes a much larger quantity of red meat than we recommend. In addition to poultry (without the skin), seafood, eggs, and white cheeses, frequently ignored foods such as sweetbreads, other organ meats, and animal brains are excellent sources of protein. These latter also contain elements needed in building the genetic chain (DNA-RNA).

A protein drink should be taken upon arising in the morning, 30 minutes before your afternoon low, and anytime you begin to feel low or cranky. It should be made with one heaping tablespoon of protein powder that contains *no* carbohydrates and that is at least 90 percent protein, one teaspoon of brewer's yeast flakes, and one-half cup of liquid such as non-cola diet sodas or one of the allowed fruit juices. Mix these ingredients thoroughly in a blender, adding several ice cubes if you wish.

Specifically *banned* from the Harper Eating Plan are: any

type of milk (because it contains lactose, a rapidly metabolized sugar); any processed meat or processed cheese; all beans except green and wax; corn; Jerusalem artichokes; peas; potatoes; rice; bananas; grapes; watermelon; apple juice; grape juice and prune juice; all refined grains (except wheat germ and unprocessed bran) as well as all products made from grains such as flour, cereal, pasta, and bread; anything containing caffeine such as cola drinks, coffee, some teas, and those pain relievers containing caffeine or other stimulants; and all alcohol with the exception of wine for cooking.

Those who are using the Eating Plan as a preventive measure may also have *unrefined* carbohydrates such as whole grain bread, corn, soy beans, and potatoes. Those people who are using the Eating Plan for regulation of glucose metabolism dysfunction can also add these unrefined carbohydrates to their diet *after* they have had one full symptom-free month on the program. These unrefined carbohydrates should be added one food at a time under the conditions stated in the full Harper Eating Plan for glucose metabolism dysfunction (appendix A).

In addition to the diet, vitamin B complex with vitamin C should be taken twice a day, two capsules each time. Each capsule should have the following formula:

Thiamin mononitrate (B1) . . . . .15 mg
Riboflavin (B2) . . . . .10 mg
Pyridoxine HCL (B3) . . . . .5 mg
Nicotinamine or niacinamide . . . . .50 mg
Pantothenic acid . . . . .10 mg
Vitamin C (ascorbic acid) . . . . 300 mg

A total of two to six tablets of amino acids plus minerals should be taken during the day. Brands which are suitable are Minamino, AG/Pro, Amino/Min and Uni-Pro 9, although a multimineral supplement must be taken with Uni-Pro 9. These should be taken according to the directions on the label. A typical formula for six tablets would be:

Protein hydrolysate (45 percent amino acids) . . . . . 50 gr
L-lysine monohydrochloride . . . . 300 mg
Di-methionine . . . . .75 mg
Iron . . . . .10 mg
Copper . . . . .1 mg

```
Iodine ....................................0.015 mg
Manganese.....................................2 mg
Potassium ...................................20 mg
Zinc .........................................2 mg
Magnesium ...................................30 mg
```
Amino acid content:
```
  Aspartic acid............................ 179 mg
  Serine .................................. 115 mg
  Glycine ................................. 107 mg
  Alanine...................................68 mg
  Arginine..................................74 mg
  Histidine ................................45 mg
  Lysine .................................. 425 mg
  Tyrosine .................................74 mg
  Tryptophan ...............................27 mg
  Phenylalanine........................... 103 mg
  Cystine ..................................16 mg
  Methionine .............................. 110 mg
  Threonine.................................84 mg
  Leucine ................................. 136 mg
  Isoleucine .............................. 101 mg
  Valine .................................. 117 mg
  Glutamic acid ........................... 226 mg
```

In addition, 400 IU (international units) of d-alpha tocopherol vitamin E should be taken daily.

Other vitamins and minerals should be taken according to individual need. A vitamin analysis can be done by computer analysis of all food intake for a week or more. This diet survey analysis gives an average daily intake of the different vitamins. This is, of course, very helpful, but it cannot accurately measure the intracellular vitamin content and whether or not each individual body is properly absorbing and utilizing the vitamins in question. It is, however, the best that can be done at the present time.

An intracellular measurement of minerals can be made through the use of the newest growth of hair at sites such as the nape of the neck. The use of hair is the most practical method. New growth of fingernails could give the same type of information, but nails grow slowly, and the part of the nail that would give the most recent information about the minerals in the body is the new growth; this would require the removal of the nail—a painful and, fortunately, unnecessary procedure.

Measuring the quantity of minerals from the bloodstream is also impractical because of the rapidity with which toxic ions are cleared from it—usually one to three days. They are deposited in various cells of the body after being removed from the bloodstream. For example, in lead toxicity the primary deposit of lead is in the bone tissue and in red cells. Even if one were to analyze the red cells, only the tip of the iceberg would be seen insofar as the total amount of lead in the body at one time is concerned.

Hair, on the other hand, is ideal for examining the various minerals present in the bloodstream. As it pierces the scalp and grows outward, the hair shaft is progressively less composed of live tissue. The new growth, therefore, will give the most recent mineral state of the body, assuming one knows how to analyze the results. The results can be used by a physician to tell in what areas supplements are needed and/or detoxification is necessary.

ALCOHOLISM

Alcoholism, while only one phase of the general problem of glucose metabolism dysfunction, has reached such gross levels of incidence in this and many other countries that it is frequently treated as a disease in and of itself. Unfortunately, this results in too little emphasis on its underlying cause and its natural control.

The dimensions of alcoholism, much like the dimensions of hypoglycemia, can never be completely measured because millions of victims do not yet know they *are* victims. The difference between "problem drinker" and "alcoholic"—confirmed dependence on alcohol—is minor though relevant; the difference between "incipient problem drinker" and "problem drinker" is much more difficult to pin down and involves millions of Americans who honestly believe they do *not* have a problem, yet guzzle at the first opportunity.

As of 1976, the number of known problem drinkers and/or alcoholics in the United States was estimated at 9 million. However, experts in the area believe that the figure is far closer to 10 percent of the population, or more than 20 million people, even though many of them would heatedly deny that they have lost control of their drinking habits.

The plague of alcoholism, as of 1976, was costing the nation almost $70 million *per day,* which is $25.5 billion per year. This daily breakdown includes at least $25.5 million in lost work production, about $23 million in health and medical costs, about $18 million in traffic accidents, $1.8 million in research and prevention programs, $1.4 million in criminal justice costs, and $400,000 in social welfare assistance.

The controversy over the origin of alcoholism has not yet been settled. Some say that it results from underlying emotional problems that a person tries to escape through drink and as a result, after a period of time, he slips into alcoholism. Others believe that the alcoholic has inherited a tendency toward the problem that is activated by the ingestion of alcohol.

In *Nutrition Against Disease,* Dr. Roger Williams points out that while most physicians associate alcoholism with malnutrition, few ever consider the possibility that it may be *caused* by malnutrition. Dr. Williams believes that it is, and he states uncategorically: *"No one who follows good nutritional practices will ever become an alcoholic."* (Emphasis added.)

The same type of position is taken by Dr. Carl Pfeiffer in *Mental and Elemental Nutrients:* "Tests have repeatedly shown that diet can affect alcoholism regardless of genetics or environment. A rat placed on a typical diet of coffee, refined foods, and soda will eventually avoid the bowl of water in his cage and selectively drink from the bowl of whisky. A diet high in carbohydrates, especially of the refined variety, can produce a drunken rat whether or not he has a mean mother or an alcoholic father"—or even a nagging mate.

The yeoman efforts of organizations such as Alcoholics Anonymous in arguing for the hourly and daily abstention from alcohol and for alcoholics to face the reality of their problem are to be commended. A lot of good comes from their sessions of self-criticism, including the confidence and self-esteem that are gained from facing the truth.

Unfortunately, however, these same groups also undermine

the very result they wish to achieve by ignoring the fact that abstinence from alcohol is removing only the symptom and does nothing to cure the disease (glucose metabolism dysfunction). At Alcoholics Anonymous meetings refined carbohydrates such as doughnuts and other pastries, as well as caffeine in the form of coffee, usually with sugar and milk added to compound the problem, are customarily served.

Alcoholics who swear off alcohol and seek refuge in other refined carbohydrates may find that they have merely exchanged one addiction for another. The flight from booze to pastries simply perpetuates the underlying problem of GMD, whose solution is found in abstaining from all refined carbohydrates, not just alcohol, as well as in nutritional supplements to establish the body's optimum function—in medical parlance, homeostasis.

The alcoholic who has given up liquor and gorged himself on other refined carbohydrates and then returns to drinking should not be regarded as merely a weak-willed derelict. Often the consumption of sweets has the effect of *increasing* the desire for alcohol—and thus the eventual return to drinking.

The real test of an alcoholic's desire to quit is whether or not he continues to follow the Harper Eating Plan after all the appropriate and correct information has been given to him.

In clinical experience, Dr. Harper has seen a very small number of alcoholics who do not have glucose metabolism dysfunction. In these cases, other solutions must be found to the problem of alcoholism.

THREE

"Heart Disease": *Public Enemy Number One*

HITTING THE JACKPOT

Cardiovascular—"heart"—disease affects almost 30 million Americans and kills 1,061,000 of these each year. Arteriosclerosis, or hardening of the arteries, is a major factor in the majority of these deaths. It is a condition so rampant that it is virtually accepted as the normal state of the body. It is the leading cause of death in white males 35 and older, the leading cause of death in black males 30 and over, the leading cause of death in black women 35 and over, and the leading cause of death in white women 40 and over.

Though common throughout all segments of the population, arteriosclerotic vascular disease affects some minorities at a rate slightly greater than for the country as a whole. This is, to a large extent, because the economically disadvantaged minorities have a higher intake of refined carbohydrates and are less likely to be taking needed vitamin and mineral supplements.

Ironically, although American Jews are usually thought of as being an "economically advantaged" group, there is also a disproportionately large amount of arteriosclerotic vascular disease in this group. There is also disproportionately more diabetes and obesity among Jews than in the surrounding population. This is probably because generations of Jews, oppressed in virtually every country, compensated at the dinner table for the oppression by characteristically and traditionally

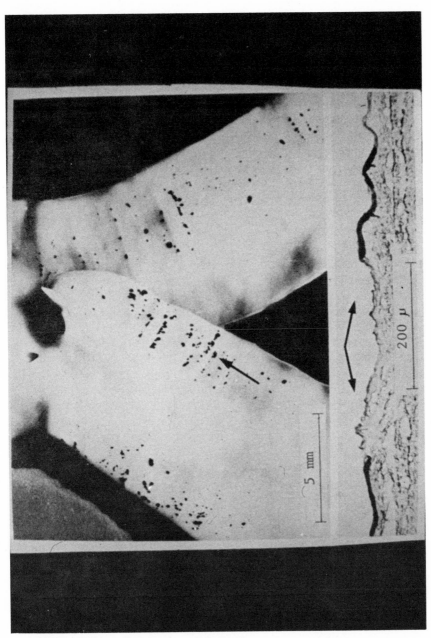

From *The Artery and the Process of Arteriosclerosis*, copyright © 1971 by Stewart Wolf

FIGURE 15

providing enormous amounts of food for family and friends, and refined carbohydrates are high on the list of typical Jewish foods.

However, arteriosclerotic vascular disease is so widespread and growing so rapidly in incidence that it is far from being the province of any one group.

Arteriosclerosis develops in a slow, insidious way, often beginning even before birth. In figure 15 we see an abdominal aorta from a stillborn infant. The stripes visible across this artery are calcium deposits that were already present at the time the child was born. Figure 16 shows a calcium stain on the femoral artery of a newborn infant. The black spots are the beginning formations of plaques. Under magnification, the black dots reveal solidified calcium already in this infant artery at birth. These extracellular and intracellular deposits lead throughout life to increasing amounts of "metastatic" calcium—that is, calcium deposited at abnormal places in the body. And calcium is the primary mineral component of most arteriosclerotic plaques.

Autopsies of infants as young as a year and a half to two years old and of young children under six have indicated that the primary cause of death was arteriosclerotic coronary artery disease! The deposits in the arteries of these infants were due to the abnormal nutrients and the vitamin D_2 ingested by the mother during pregnancy that crossed the placenta during the gestation period.

The only type of vitamin D that is needed by man is D_3, which is produced in the body as a result of exposure of the melanin-producing cells of the skin to sunlight. It is also available from fish liver oil. All other forms of vitamin D, including D_2, which is used to "enrich" or "fortify" milk and other foods, are not necessary and, like D_2, may be harmful to man. Vitamin D_2 has been linked to the deposit of calcium in the heart valves of children, and for this reason it was outlawed in Germany over 50 years ago. Vitamin D_2 should be avoided by pregnant women in order to avoid the deposit of calcium in abnormal locations, including heart valves and and arteries of their unborn children.

Bear in mind that for arteriosclerotic plaques to form there must be a fatty matrix to which the calcium and other minerals attach themselves. The arteriosclerotic buildup begins with the junk food consumed by the mother and continues

84

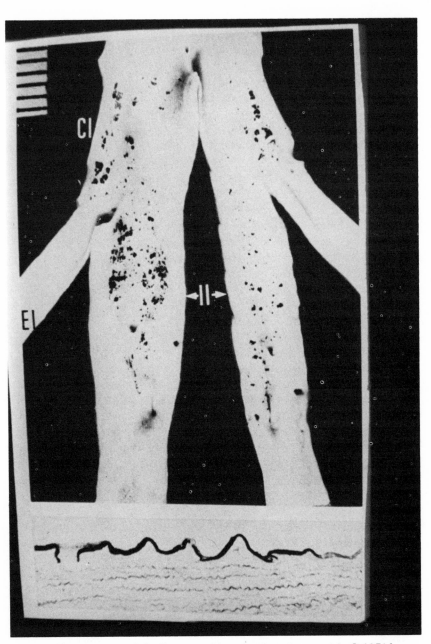

FIGURE 16

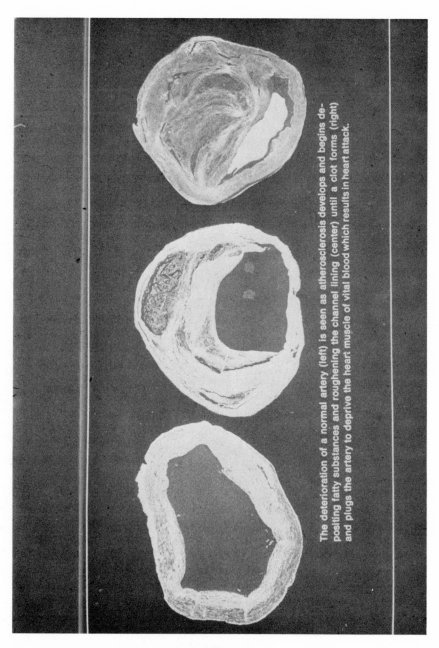

The deterioration of a normal artery (left) is seen as atherosclerosis develops and begins depositing fatty substances and roughening the channel lining (center) until a clot forms (right) and plugs the artery to deprive the heart muscle of vital blood which results in heart attack.

FIGURE 17

with the junk food consumed by the child. The development is slow, subtle, and certain.

In figure 17 we see the typical advance of arteriosclerosis in an individual who lives in a polluted environment, including the pollution which he himself creates. Figure 18 shows a plaque taken from the abdominal aorta of a 72-year-old man. This is what clogs our arteries! The small pinpoint in the center is the channel through which this man's entire blood supply for his pelvis and legs must pass. Notice the winglike objects on the plaques. They are deposits of calcium and other minerals such as lead, mercury, and copper as well as other polluting chemicals that are acquired from air, water, and food sources.

Our circulatory system is not a great deal different from the plumbing system found in the average home. If a water pipe in your home breaks or becomes plugged, it will *not* be where

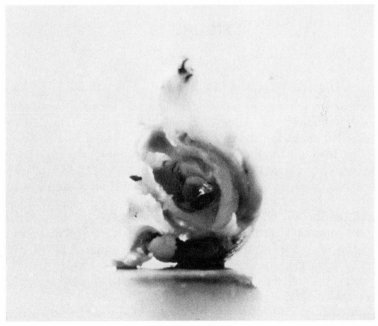

FIGURE 18

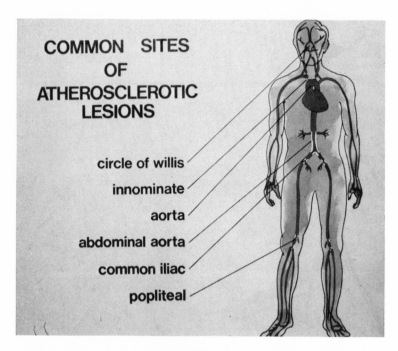

FIGURE 19

the water was moving in a straight line. The break or disruption always occurs at a curve or joint or where a large pipe joins a smaller one. At those places there will be a buildup of corroded material. Minerals and acids present in the fluids going through the pipes will be precipitated on the pipe itself by eddying currents caused by the passage of fluids through the branches. In just the same way, we find plaquing anywhere larger arteries branch into smaller arteries, arterioles, and capillaries. Thus, as can be seen in figure 19, some of the most common sites for plaquing are at the Circle of Willis and in the abdomen at the branching of the renal arteries, the junction of the abdominal aorta and the iliac, which goes to the pelvis and legs, and in the legs at the branching of the femoral artery.

The final result of years of abuse of one's body that results in arterial plaquing may be a "heart attack," when the coronary artery is so blocked that the blood flow to the heart muscle is reduced or stopped, or a "stroke," where the blood supply and the oxygen it carries to the brain is reduced or stopped.

Of the about 700,000 people who have heart attacks each year, more than half never reach the hospital alive. Unfortunately, the average heart attack victim procrastinates for three or more hours before attempting to get help, even when he experiences the typical symptoms of a heart attack. This may be due to the fact that the majority of victims do not even realize that they have had cardiovascular disease for years, and therefore, when they do have a heart attack, they misinterpret the symptoms.

Symptoms of cardiovascular disease occur only late in its development—when approximately *70 percent* of the body's ability to circulate blood has been lost. A potential heart attack victim can visit his doctor, have a complete physical examination including an electrocardiogram, be told he is "healthy as a horse," walk out into the street and drop dead of a heart attack.

In fact, the expression "healthy as a horse" is itself a dodge: horses, as well as other domesticated animals, frequently have heart attacks, heart disease, diabetes, and even cancer, while animals that live in the wild do not. Animals subsisting on a natural diet in their natural habitats are remarkably free from degenerative diseases, while those kept and fed by man are not.

While arteriosclerosis due to years of building plaque formations is the major contributor to heart attacks, there are also other factors that contribute to a "vascular catastrophe." The relation of all these factors can be seen in figure 20. Most important among these is excessive and/or continual emotional stress. But while stress is important, it is not always easy to determine what will be a stressful situation. Studies have indicated, for example, that men with higher positions in business, higher salaries and more responsibility have *fewer* heart attacks than do employees in lower brackets. On the other hand, the turmoil caused by making a major change in one's lifestyle such as a change in jobs or a move to a new community seems to be the kind of stress that affects potential heart attack victims.

VASCULAR CATASTROPHIES

CAUSES & CONTRIBUTING FACTORS

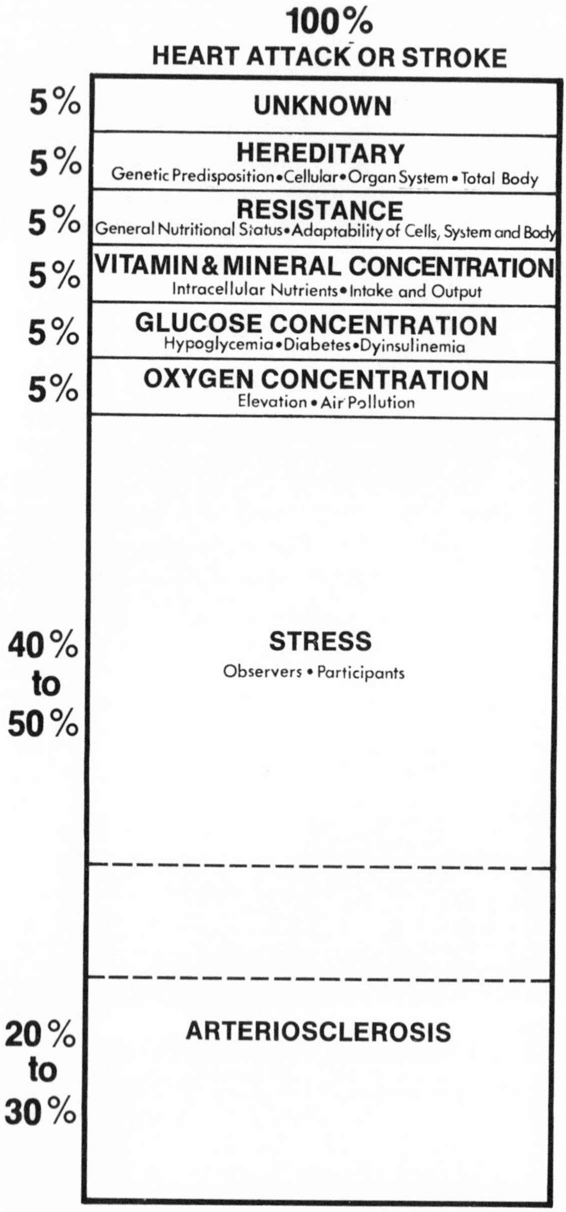

100%

HEART ATTACK OR STROKE

5%	**UNKNOWN**
5%	**HEREDITARY** Genetic Predisposition•Cellular•Organ System • Total Body
5%	**RESISTANCE** General Nutritional Status•Adaptability of Cells, System and Body
5%	**VITAMIN & MINERAL CONCENTRATION** Intracellular Nutrients•Intake and Output
5%	**GLUCOSE CONCENTRATION** Hypoglycemia•Diabetes•Dyinsulinemia
5%	**OXYGEN CONCENTRATION** Elevation • Air Pollution
40% **to** **50%**	**STRESS** Observers • Participants
20% **to** **30%**	**ARTERIOSCLEROSIS**

FIGURE 20

The concentration of oxygen is another important factor in vascular catastrophes. If oxygen availability is reduced because of high altitudes or urban air pollution or one's own pollution of the air by smoking, the body will not be able to get enough oxygen in the bloodstream to transfer to the cells. At this point the individual involved is well on the way to heart disease. Shortness of breath and, in some cases, chest pain (angina) are symptoms that occur in the absence of an adequate oxygen supply to the cells of the body.

Physical exercise, or in most cases the lack of it, is also important in heart disease. There is an increased efficiency of the heart in pumping blood and withstanding physical stress when exercise is done on a regular basis. Unfortunately, watching television does not qualify as physical exercise. Americans spend more than 50 percent of their leisure time in this occupation; we spend less than one percent of leisure time in physical exercise, and the great majority of us have no physical exercise during our working hours.

Dietary considerations are also involved in vascular catastrophes. In addition to the part it plays in the formation of arteriosclerotic plaques, junk food also causes vitamin and mineral deficiencies and leads to obesity, which of course places an additional strain on the heart as well as other organs.

Rarely, however, are Americans deprived of an adequate number of *calories*. In fact, we are probably the most *overfed* and at the same time *undernourished* industrial society in the world today.

The problem is not the amount of fuel taken into the body but rather the quality of the fuel consumed. We would not consider using only gasoline to operate an automobile: we need oil in the crank case, transmission fluid in the transmission, brake fluid in the brake cylinders, water in the radiator, and air in the tires. Similarly, we cannot operate our bodies, which are infinitely more complicated than an automobile, on calories alone. A balanced diet of protein, fat, and carbohydrates, as well as air, water, vitamins, and minerals, is required.

An automobile owner should not use high-octane aviation gasoline in a low power automobile engine because it would overheat the engine and cause a malfunction. Neither should we expect to place "high octane" refined carbohydrates in our bodies and expect them to operate without malfunctions.

It is interesting to note that Americans spend more money on preventive maintenance for their automobiles than they spend on preventive health maintenance for their own bodies.

The time one is most likely to suffer a vascular catastrophe is when one's blood sugar is low. Glucose tolerance tests run at hourly intervals around the clock indicate that blood sugar levels will most often be at their lowest point—perhaps low enough that the heart and/or brain cannot get sufficient oxygen and glucose—several hours after going to bed. By the time the person realizes something is wrong, contacts an ambulance unit and is on the way to the hospital, it is close to 3:00 A.M.—the prime time for the arrival of the vascular catastrophe patient in emergency rooms of hospitals across the country. Note that it is not when the victim is actively engaged in physical stress that most heart attacks or strokes occur.

Some 40 percent of heart attack victims die as a result of their first heart attack. The most critical time for a heart attack victim is within the first hour after the attack. Delays in locating the doctor, stopping to pack a suitcase, or indecisiveness can be the difference between life and death. It is crucial that the victim be taken to the nearest emergency room available as quickly as possible.

The second most critical period of time for a heart attack victim is the week immediately following an attack. If a person survives the first week he has probably won the first round, and he can take steps to head off another attack.

Prolonged and oppressive pain or unusual discomfort in the *center* of the chest is one of the warning signs of a heart attack. It is a popular misconception that this pain will radiate to the shoulder and arm. It *may,* but it need not. Pain occurring with a heart attack most often is located in the center of the chest or very close to the actual location of the heart. Sweating may accompany the pain, and nausea, vomiting, and shortness of breath may also occur.

More than 1,800,000 people have strokes every year in this country, and more than 270,000 die from them. The warning signs that a stroke may be occurring are sudden, temporary weakness or numbness of the face, arms, or legs; a temporary loss of speech or trouble in speaking or understanding speech or difficulty in word association and in completing sentences;

temporary blindness or diminution of vision, usually in one eye rather than both; episodes of double vision; unexplained dizziness or unsteadiness.

The unfortunate thing is that many of these fatal strokes could have been prevented by properly taking care of the hypertension (high blood pressure) that preceded them. More than 10 percent of all Americans (about 24,000,000) are hypertensive. About half of those who have the problem do not know they have it, and 25 percent of those who do know they have it are not doing anything about it. The remaining 25 percent know they have it and are trying to do something about it but only half of them (12.5 percent of the total number of hypertensives) are being successful in controlling the state. (See figure 21.) The result of this lack of control of high blood pressure is often death. Hypertensives are three to five times more likely to be victims of heart attacks or heart failure or strokes as well as of other problems such as kidney failure.

THE COMMON APPROACH

Tragically, the most common "treatment" for heart disease in this country is the one in which the physician simply observes the patient until it is time to call the mortician. While observing patients with arteriosclerosis, these physicians often say such things as: "Well, you've got to die some day." "It's a condition of aging." "There's nothing I can do about it." "Come back in a month and have your blood pressure taken." "Learn to live with it."

The second most common therapy for ateriosclerotic vascular disease is the use of arterial dilating agents, such as nitroglycerine, peritrate, cyclospasmol, and the like. The trouble with dilating agents is that they work well in a normal artery, but not very well in an arteriosclerotic one. A rubber tube can be dilated easily, but a lead pipe cannot be dilated without breaking—and a clogged, blocked, arteriosclerotic artery is more like a lead pipe than a rubber tube.

AWARENESS & THERAPY
OF 23 MILLION PERSONS
IN THE UNITED STATES
WITH HIGH BLOOD PRESSURE

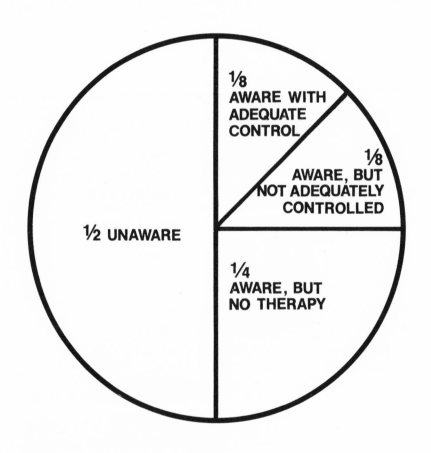

SOURCE: estimated by National Heart & Lung Institute

FIGURE 21

Dilating agents are at best a temporary crutch, for they only dilate the undiseased straight segments of the affected artery. Their use may, for example, help alleviate angina pains, but they do not clear up or control arteriosclerosis, which is not, after all, a segmental disease. It occurs throughout the entire body.

The third most common therapy for the treatment of heart disease is cardiac or vascular surgery that is done in any of a variety of ingenious ways (such as transplanting a portion of the leg veins into the chest cavity), all at a cost of anywhere from $22,000 to $38,000.

As Dr. Berman points out in *The Solid Gold Stethoscope,*

> The new answer to one of the biggest killers in medical history may yet become the biggest killing in medical economics. Though the 'bypass' for coronary heart disease is similar to the one discarded twenty years ago, it's now back by popular demand and doing a landoffice business. It has not been conclusively proved yet, but then neither has aspirin—and billions of dollars worth of that little moneymaker has already been sold. If tens of thousands of patients believe and are waiting—who among those altruistic, reticent, selfless cardiac surgeons is going to disillusion them?

Whether a patient survives such surgery depends as much on which surgeon or surgical team he sees as on how competent that surgeon or team is. Some physicians will not consider cardiovascular surgery until the disease has reached an extreme degree of severity. Others will operate at the drop of a hat. Obviously the condition of the patient at the time of surgery will have an important effect on the recovery (or lack of it) of the patient.

Dr. Harper attended a cardiovascular conference given by the American College of Cardiology in 1975 at which some of the most recent "thinking" about cardiovascular surgery and the techniques used to get a patient on the operating table in the least amount of time was presented. Among the new approaches is a system in Spokane, Washington, in which every patient who complains of chest pains is rushed to a central hospital. Radio calls for the cardiovascular team are dispatched from the ambulance and things are so organized that within five minutes of the patient's arrival at the hospital he is in the cardiopulmonary lab. Within 30 minutes of his arrival the patient has had a coronary angiogram, which is an X-ray examination of the arteries of the heart. Within an hour of arrival, the patient is on the operating table, with chest shaved and scrubbed, release forms signed, and ready for the surgeon. Thus, every citizen in Spokane who complained of chest pain and who was rushed through this novel system was operated on and a coronary bypass was performed within two and a half hours after arrival in the emergency room.

Dr. Harper was told that solely on the basis of an abnormal angiogram and complaint of chest pain, surgery costing more than $20,000 is performed. The problem with this is that virtually every man and woman over age 45 in this country is going to have an abnormal angiogram, and that chest pains, even on the left side of the chest, may also occur with bronchitis, pneumonia, pulmonary embolism, gallbladder disease, and ulcers. Such pain does not occur only during a heart attack. In addition, there is no confirmatory evidence of a heart attack (such as heart enzyme level elevation) for several hours and sometimes for as long as two to three days after an attack. Electrocardiograms (EKGs, the graphic recordings of electrical impulses produced by the heart) may or may not be abnormal immediately after an attack. Yet an abnormal EKG or angiogram is the standard used to justify surgery in the Spokane program. And the *surgery* itself may change the EKG from normal to abnormal: the severance of muscle fiber of the heart causes a scar to form, and this process itself is a form of surgically induced heart attack.

When the speaker was questioned by Dr. Harper, it was learned that scare tactics had been used on the patients and the patients' families to get their signatures on the forms giving consent for surgery. Such statements as "He might not live until morning if we don't operate now" or "He's in a bad way; it's surgery or death—take your choice," were common.

A word to the wise would seem to be that if you ever have chest pain in Spokane, don't tell anyone; just take the first train, bus, or airplane out of the city.

Unfortunately, at that same conference there were physicians from all sections of the country who wanted to know how they could set up such an "efficient" system in their home cities.

Coronary artery surgery has become the "in" way to deal with heart disease, and it has been widely promoted by medical groups and the media. But, at best, it is risky. In *The Un-*

kindest Cut Marcia Millman writes: "There is clear evidence that the operation itself may cause significant damage to the heart, contains many long-term risks and actually accelerates the progression of coronary artery disease."

Estimates by medical economists are that 80,000 cases of coronary artery bypass surgery, costing $3 billion, were performed in 1976, and the projections are that this rapidly growing field may over the next 10 years become a $100 billion a year industry dominating the nation's health budget and, parenthetically, utilizing millions of dollars in sophisticated electronics gadgetry produced by the technology-electronics-computer industry, which has moved from warfare and space technology to the health field.

In coronary bypass surgery (saphenous vein coronary artery surgery) the plugged-up (occluded) parts of the three main coronary arteries that transport blood to the heart muscle are "bypassed" by the insertion of grafts made from veins taken from the legs. These grafts are inserted between the distal ends of the coronary arteries and the aorta (the largest artery in the body) to detour blood around the occluded areas.

Ideally, this procedure is supposed to be effective in reducing the awesome chest pain (angina pectoris) that is sometimes present in heart disease, in preventing heart attacks and the deterioration of the heart muscle, in prolonging life and in helping the patient withstand more physical activity. The operation does relieve angina pain in 85 percent of the cases at least temporarily, but some physicians insist that this can be done in more cases (95 percent) *without* surgery. As for the other goals of bypass surgery, they are even less likely to justify the surgery.

What most heart patients unfortunately do not know as they are wheeled into the operating room is that the surgery itself is in no way a cure. At best it is a short-term palliative procedure for which there is no hard evidence that it either prevents heart attacks or prolongs life. In fact, there is growing statistical evidence that it may actually enhance the chances of a heart attack, since myocardial infarction (heart attack) occurs in anywhere from 5 to 40 percent of patients *during* or immediately after coronary artery surgery, depending on who is doing the counting. The number of deaths during or immediately thereafter is between 7 and 12 percent of the patients.

97

Almost as bad, some reports indicate that up to 30 percent of the vein grafts themselves become blocked or occluded within one year after surgery, and one study indicates that the insertion of grafts increases the likelihood that new, total occlusions will develop in the arteries before and after the site of the graft insertions.

R. S. Ross of the Cardiovascular Disease Division of the Department of Medicine, Johns Hopkins Hospital, concluded in "Ischemic Heart Disease" that bypass surgery has not been shown to increase a person's life expectancy or to reduce his chance of having a heart attack.

The prognosis for bypass surgery is not encouraging.

THE UNCOMMON APPROACH: MAN'S MIRACLE MOLECULE

In addition to the orthodox ways of dealing with heart disease enumerated above, there is an unorthodox therapy that has nothing to do with dilating agents or surgery and that is saving lives and eliminating suffering in people who might otherwise spend the rest of their lives in a rest home.

This therapy is called chelation (kee-LAY-shun), from the Greek word for claw. It "claws out" the toxic mineral deposits in the circulatory system by chemically binding with the minerals in such a way that they become soluble and are removed from the body through the kidneys.

Vitamins E and C are themselves natural chelating agents and so are the amino acids. They perform some chelating functions, but they are not strong enough to work in the therapeutic management of vascular disease. Other chemicals have much more affinity for the unwanted minerals in the circulatory system. One of these was discovered in Germany in 1931 and was introduced in this country in 1941 by Dr. Frederick Bursworth, a biochemist at Georgetown Medical School.

The drug, ethylene-diamene-tetracetic acid, or EDTA for short, was licensed to Abbott Laboratories and primary animal research studies were performed at several research centers in the United States. It was approved by the FDA as a chelating agent to remove heavy minerals such as lead from the body. Dr. Norman E. Clarke, Sr., a cardiologist at Providence Hospital in Detroit, observed in the treatment of battery factory workers for lead poisoning that the treated patients began to report alleviation of their symptoms of chest pain, intermittent claudication (pain in the large muscles of the leg due to lack of oxygen carried by the arterial system), and an increase in the patients' feelings of well-being and exercise tolerance.

Dr. Clarke, still very active in his late seventies, wrote several papers on the subject and has been credited as having been the first to use it on human beings in this country. He is also hailed as a chelation pioneer by the Soviet Union, where chelation therapy is the second most common form of treatment for arteriosclerotic vascular disease. It is the preferred modality of treatment in Czechoslovakia.

Dr. Clarke found that nine out of ten patients treated with chelation therapy for angina pain experienced relief. This study was reported extensively in the medical literature. It was later found that up to three months following the therapy mineral deposits *continued* to be excreted from the body. And the arteries became softer as the minerals continued to be removed.

As late as January 8, 1970, the Food and Drug Administration referred to calcium or disodium EDTA as follows: "This drug is possibly effective in occlusive vascular disorders and the treatment of pathologic conditions to which calcium tissue deposits or hyper-calcemia may contribute other than those listed above." In other words, as late as January, 1970, the FDA recognized and approved the use of EDTA in vascular disease. But then the FDA changed its position, *not* because tests have found the substance to be unsafe, but for political and bureaucratic reasons.

The problem was that the patents held by Abbott Laboratories on EDTA ran out after the Food, Drug and Cosmetic Act was amended in 1962 so that substances that had previously been required only to show that they were safe now had to be shown to be safe *and* effective. Since the patents on EDTA ran out and any drug company could then produce the substance, it was not worth the great amount of time and expense to relicense the drug under the provisions of the new law. So, since EDTA remains "licensed" only for use in lead poisoning, its use in treating heart disease technically makes it an "unproven remedy" under FDA regulations. EDTA is still produced and is increasingly being used in heart disease, but it is not sanctioned by the FDA or the AMA for such use.

The political and economic opposition to EDTA is more subtle and complex. The use of EDTA is far less expensive than surgery and other modalities used in the treatment of heart disease. As compared to placing one's life in the hands of a surgical team that may involve up to a dozen people, treatment with EDTA is comparatively simple, if time consuming, for it merely involves intravenous infusion of the material into the bloodstream during a period of several hours.

To understand how EDTA works, note that the heavy toxic minerals—calcium, lead, mercury, copper, and others—are divalent, all having a 2+ positive charge. They are deposited in a layer of fat, cholesterol, and phospholipids or in the arterial walls.

The cholesterol, fats, and phospholipids are the result of consuming carbohydrates that the body is unable to assimilate, metabolize, and utilize. Avoiding cholesterol in food is not as beneficial in treating heart disease as has been claimed. Cholesterol is produced by the body and is essential to its proper functioning. It is bad only when it appears in arterial plaques. Eliminating cholesterol from one's diet merely eliminates many foods of high nutritional value. It does not lower the cholesterol level of the body since the body simply produces more cholesterol to make up the difference. A totally carbohydrate-free diet, even when it is high in cholesterol, will reduce cholesterol levels.

In fact, cholesterol is not the primary problem. It is simply a substance that the body manufactures and uses to store energy in the bloodstream. The cholesterol molecule is small, measuring about two or three microns. The molecules of the fatty substances called triglycerides, on the other hand, measure 18 to 25 microns. They are too large to easily traverse the body's system of tiny capillaries, and so may clog up the small arteries, causing a damming effect and thus depriving tissue of the oxygen and glucose that it should be getting.

EDTA, which could be described as "man's miracle molecule," has the unique capacity of donating from each of its six carbon atoms an electron that "binds" a divalent mineral and holds it in place—hence the description of chelation therapy as "mineral- and metal-binding." It is a biochemical reaction in which EDTA, a synthetic amino acid, as it traverses the arterial wall, combines with the molecules of a harmful mineral. The reaction changes the mineral from a solid to a liquid, which is passed out of the body through the kidneys. The amount that is being passed out can be measured in the urine.

The process is much the same as that which takes place when table salt is dissolved in water. When salt combines with water it changes from a solid to a liquid that cannot be seen. All chelating agents—vitamin E, natural amino acids, EDTA—work in a similar way, "binding," or liquefying, minerals so they can be excreted from the body.

As the mineral molecules are eliminated from the body, the pressure of the bloodstream moving through the arteries works in a manner similar to holding a hose on a spot on a wall: if you hold the hose on the spot long enough, the water pressure will loosen the dirt and the spot will disappear. In an artery, the pressure and eddying currents break down the molecules of fat, cholesterol, and phospholipids and wash them into the bloodstream to the liver, which then excretes them into the digestive track and clears the body of many of the accumulations of toxic minerals within the arterial system.

Another primary action of chelating agents is to remove toxic minerals—particularly lead, cadmium, and mercury—from the walls and membranes of cells. The lysosome, a membrane within a membrane, is the "toilet" for individual cells. It is contained within the protoplasm of the cell. Mitochondria are tiny "manufacturing plants" that occur within each cell. As the mitochondria produce enzymes, which are activated by the trace minerals and other products of metabolism, toxic minerals may accumulate on the lysosome, thus reducing cellular efficiency, a process that increases as we become older.

This buildup is similar to what would happen at a manufacturing plant if the boxes in which raw materials arrive were simply tossed out a window into the parking lot. The parking lot would soon be filled with empty boxes, byproducts of the plant's manufacturing activity.

When EDTA enters the cell, it combines with the "left-over" minerals that have been deposited on the lysosome, and they are excreted from the cell, thus increasing the efficiency of the cell's mitochondria and, consequently, increasing the overall efficiency of the cell.

The process of lipid peroxidation (breakdown) of the outer cellular membrane causes deterioration of the membrane and allows vital nutrients to escape from the cell. Lipid peroxidation of the cellular membrane is brought about by the accumulation of liquid-state divalent minerals within the membrane. The more minerals that accumulate in the cellular membrane, the greater the breakdown. EDTA binds these minerals, removing them from the cellular membrane and thus protecting it from their effects.

The units of the cellular membrane are also protected or held intact by the action of vitamin E and selenium, a trace mineral. Selenium is a two-edged sword. Small amounts are necessary for the maintenance of the cellular membrane, but excessive amounts may become toxic to the body's cells. The actions of vitamin C enhance and are synergistic with vitamin E activity, and thus are necessary to the body.

A final primary action of EDTA is to bind the free (ionic) calcium in the bloodstream, hence lowering serum calcium levels. Two forms of calcium are present in the blood: a protein-linked calcium complex and an ionic form that is not linked to protein. EDTA will not bind the protein-complex calcium, and thus this type of calcium, which is the type in bone tissue, is retained in the body. It is the ionic form that is bound to the EDTA molecule and removed from the bloodstream, thus lowering the serum calcium level. Activation of the parathyroid glands (the tiny pea-sized glands behind the thyroid gland) takes place when the serum calcium level is lowered and parathormone is secreted, which in turn releases the calcium from plaques, joints, et cetera, into the bloodstream. This release of metastatic calcium raises the serum calcium level so that the state of optimum metabolic function within the organism (homeostasis) occurs.

Many scientists unfamiliar with the metabolic processes and homeostatic mechanisms of the "calcium pool" have criticized chelation therapy because of their mistaken belief that EDTA might attack the calcium in the bones and thus lower this mineral content. However, instead of bone-thinning or calcium loss, in elderly patients (in whom bones have demineralized) there is an increased calcium deposit within the bones after EDTA treatment.

102

There are 21 different demonstrated or postulated effects of EDTA within the body, and the scientific literature on chelation therapy is extensive: more than 1,700 articles on the subject have been printed in English alone. Yet what we often encounter is that the patient with whom we discuss chelation therapy for, say, angina pain will go to the average cardiologist or family physician and ask about it and be told that there is no real evidence of the therapy's positive effects and that it might even be toxic. The fact is that known toxicity levels for EDTA itself are extremely low: the LD50 (lethal dose for 50 percent of test animals) is 2,000 milligrams per kilo as compared with 60 per kilo for aspirin. However, the toxicity may vary depending on the toxic mineral being passed through the kidneys. The chelation of calcium carries the least toxicity, while the toxicity of mercury chelation is more than 200 times greater.

The statement that there is no real evidence to support the benefits of chelation therapy is a gross falsehood. However, it is one which is accepted not only by Establishment medicine, but also by the federal government, in spite of the fact that EDTA was at one time recognized as "possibly effective in occlusive vascular disorders." When this acceptance and quasi recommendation was withdrawn, chelation was "wished away" and in some states "legislated away." There is simply no economic advantage to hospitals, thoracic surgeons, anesthesiologists, or the pharmaceutical and medical industry in chelation therapy programs.

Chelation therapy is a relatively inexpensive procedure (especially when compared to one alternative, bypass surgery) that can be performed by any general practitioner or internist with adequate clinical facilities and a practical working knowledge of the therapeutic applications.

Chelation should be seen as only a part, albeit a central part, of a total metabolic or holistic approach to the problem of heart disease. The total program involves a radical change in lifestyle, especially in the area of eating habits: the diet of refined carbohydrates which did so much to contribute to the problem in the first place must be replaced with biologically sound eating habits. In addition, vitamin and mineral supplements based on individual needs must be added, the continual stress one lives with must be minimized as much as possible, and a reasonable exercise program must be undertaken to prevent a recurrence of the cardiovascular problem.

Chelation therapy is often chosen as an alternative to surgery. This was true in the case of Dr. R. G., a physicist and college administrator. He had suffered two heart attacks and was unable to function without frequent angina. Heart surgery was recommended to him, but he decided to seek alternatives and eventually went to Louisiana to receive 15 chelation treatments from a physician practicing there. His angina rapidly disappeared, but since he had been declared totally disabled by a major cardiac rehabilitation center, getting reinstated to his college job was a bit of a problem: the school officials could not understand how he could function.

Dr. R. G. has received an additional 40 treatments through the years in order to sustain normal cardiac function and to keep his blood pressure normal. He is presently on an exercise program of running, jogging, walking, and bicycling. He has sustained no further episodes of angina since his original treatment, and his cardiac functions have remained normal. His exercise tolerance on a stress EKG has progressed steadily. After his original heart attack he was able to last only six minutes at a 10-degree angle on a stress treadmill; now he is able to endure 15 minutes at 14 degrees without changes in his electrocardiogram.

Dr. R. G. is now fully employed and functional. He continues on an eating program with supplementary minerals and an adequate exercise program to maintain a healthy state and to prevent or delay a redevelopment of arteriosclerosis.

At the age of 65, H. D. experienced a coronary occlusion on a trip to Lake Tahoe, in an area with an elevation of more than 5,000 feet where oxygen concentration in the air is lower than at sea level. Upon admission to a hospital he was found to have elevated blood pressure and electrocardiogram and enzyme functions compatible with damage to the heart muscle.

When he was discharged from the hospital he was given an antihypertensive medication to lower his blood pressure, a diuretic to eliminate excess fluids from the body and to lower his blood pressure, and a sedative to help him sleep at night. In addition, he was given nitroglycerine to be used to fight the angina attacks that resulted from an inadequate delivery of oxygen to the heart. Between the time of his heart attack and April 3, 1974, when he consulted Dr. Harper about the possibility of chelation therapy, he averaged five to ten nitroglycerine tablets a day. After laboratory tests determined that he was a suitable candidate for chelation, he began to receive infusions intravenously with a chelating agent three times a week, beginning April 15, 1974. By the end of the tenth treatment, H. D.'s chest pain was no longer present, and there was no longer any need for the nitroglycerine tablets. When he completed 21 treatments on May 31, 1974, he experienced minor chest pains on exertion and occasionally at night while lying prone. An additional nine treatments were given, beginning June 5, 1974, which resulted in marked improvement in his vascular system.

Foods high in calcium and refined carbohydrates had been removed from H. D.'s diet and high doses of vitamin B6 and B complex were administered during the entire time of his chelation treatments. An exercise program was begun on June 4, 1974, and by the end of August he was able to walk both up and down hills on a program of an increase in pulse to 100 beats a minute or until the beginning of chest pain. He experienced no chest pain during the two intervening months. By the end of September he was able to walk two miles a day, do extensive yard work (including using a hand mower), and carry cement bags. No medication or chemicals other than vitamins were prescribed.

In April, 1975, H. D. noticed the onset of minor arthritic pains in the elbow and some to the front of the chest. He had not been using nitroglycerine for more than a year. He had been walking three-and-a-half miles a day for more than a month. After receiving five additional chelation treatments, his exercise was increased to walking four miles a day.

In February, 1976, an additional five treatments were administered in order to maintain more adequately functioning cells and increased circulatory volume to the entire cardiovascular system. H. D.'s progress has continued with proper eating habits and active exercise.

In February, 1977, H. D. was rechecked. He was walking four miles a day and doing fifteen knee bends and several other calisthenic exercises for 30 minutes a day including a cardiac exercise for breathing. He had not experienced any chest pains since December, 1975. Now, at the age of 70, he continues to experience an active, enthusiastic retirement with a normal electrocardiogram and maintenance of blood pressure levels that are normal for a much younger man.

For several months, A. G., a 59-year-old advertising executive, had been experiencing what he described as a crushing weight on his chest during any type of exercise. An angiogram performed in November, 1974, showed coronary artery disease with complete blockage of one vessel.

A. G. rejected surgery and began a nutritional program that gave him a little improvement in his condition. He then learned about chelation therapy from a friend and presented himself to Dr. Harper for treatment in March, 1976.

Although A. G.'s angiogram showed marked abnormality, his electrocardiograms had remained normal. His exercise tolerance was minimal before the onset of chest pain.

After laboratory analysis and X-ray examinations to ascertain that there was normal kidney, liver, and lung function, the patient embarked on a course of chelation therapy between October, 1976, and December, 1976. The treatment program was comprised of the infusion of a chelating fluid including EDTA three times a week and a nutritional program. A. G.'s angina pains diappeared after only a few treatments, and his blood pressure and other data remained normal.

By the middle of February, 1977, A. G. was able to participate in very strenuous mountain hiking and reported amazing endurance. He was working very productively and his ability to think and coordinate thought had improved.

The patient experienced minor chest pain after two miles of running or after brisk walking for two miles followed by one mile of running. A. G. participated in a Sierra Club hike for seven hours over a six-mile course uphill without experiencing chest pain. He now hikes two times a week in addition to his normal occupational duties.

Since his treatment A. G. has continued on a prescribed nutritional program, and it is believed that he will remain in a normal state of health by maintaining a normal nutritional intake and adequate exercise for the rest of his life.

Chelation therapy has been criticized because it is said that the effects are not always permanent. However, no treatment is permanent, and chelation has the advantage that, as indicated in the cases just described, should a patient have the need, he may be re-treated with no risk of death or morbidity. On the other hand, surgery, as they say, is "once done, always done." It cannot be undone.

No matter what modality is used to treat a patient with heart disease, the most long-lasting effects are brought about by that which only the patient can do: a change in lifestyle, including a nutritional program and an adequate exercise program. This is also the key to an even better "treatment": the *prevention* of heart disease.

One of the ways to measure the efficacy of an individual's circulatory system is with a system called thermography, which shows the heat patterns in the body. Since heat is produced in the body as a result of cell metabolism, which can only take place in the presence of oxygen (delivered to the various parts of the body by the circulatory system), thermography indirectly measures arterial blood circulation. The warmest areas in the body show up as the lightest in a thermogram and consequently reflect those parts of the body that must be receiving an adequate supply of oxygen via the circulatory system. The areas in which the circulatory system is less efficient will show up as darker or colder on the thermogram.

Because cancer cells metabolize—that is, engage in chemical activity—at a higher rate than do surrounding cells, thus producing a lighter, or hotter, "spot" on the thermogram, thermography is also a useful tool in the early detection of breast cancer, and it has the added advantage of being completely safe even in repeated usage. X-ray, including mammography (the most common method used in detecting breast cancer), can itself become a *cause* of cancer when used repeatedly.

By taking photographs of the heat patterns in the body as shown in thermography, we can compare the patterns in a patient over a period of time. Figure 22 shows an individual prior to any treatment. Figure 23 shows the same patient after 30 chelation treatments. Increasing cell metabolism is clearly shown by the growth of light areas in the series of photographs, which were all taken under identical conditions to eliminate variables of heat in the body. Since this metabolism is possible only because of the increased amount of oxygen in those areas, the photographs also indirectly show a vastly improved circulatory system.

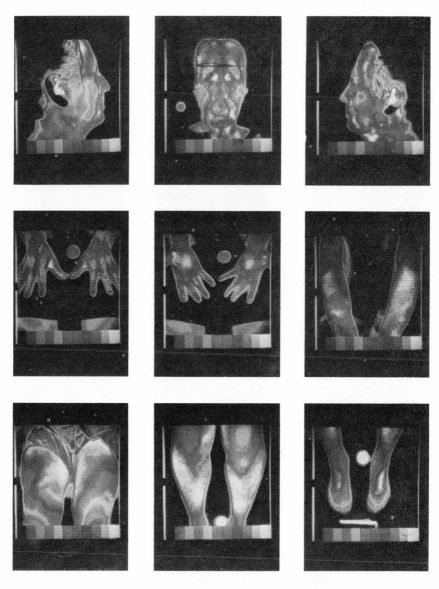

FIGURE 22

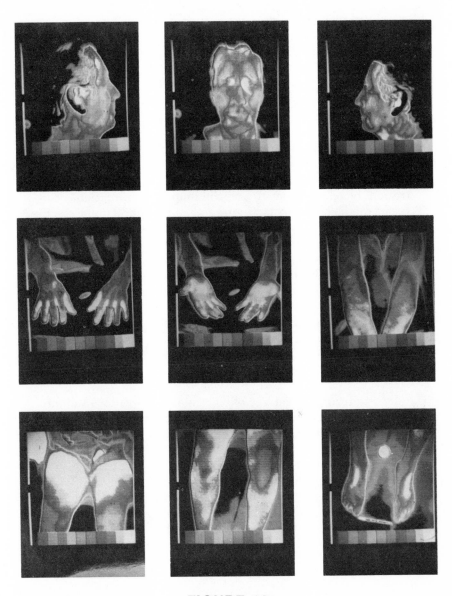

FIGURE 23

BEATING HEART DISEASE
THE NATURAL WAY

We have pointed to nutritional factors as constituting one of the most important elements in arterial disorders, and to arteriosclerosis and stress as the primary causes of heart disease. In fact, stress may be the single biggest contributing factor in heart disease, with arteriosclerosis being equal or a close second. Other important factors include oxygen concentration, blood sugar level, and the immediate nutritional status of the body in terms of vitamins and minerals and resistance built up by exercise—or the lack of it, which contributes markedly to the development of a vascular catastrophe.

The extent to which hereditary factors may influence or predispose our bodies to heart disease is not known, but it is an element that remains regardless of the care or abuse with which we treat our bodies.

In the anatomy of a vascular catastrophe, note in figure 20 (page 90) the change in percentages that occurs when one factor or another increases or decreases, depending upon individual responses.

In our technological society no one is going to eliminate stress by waving a magic wand: it is a part of our urban environment. But one may adjust to it, learn to cope with it, and change those behavioral patterns which emanate from it. So long as problems of stress are handled early in life and a lifestyle minimizing the effects of it are adopted, even nutritional abuse may not result in vascular catastrophes until one is well advanced in years. We know this from studying peoples who are less advanced and more rural than we are, who also have dangerous eating habits, but who have nowhere near the level of heart disease and other degenerative diseases that Western man suffers.

Inasmuch as eating habits are an important element in the development of heart disease, how much we eat and what we eat become primary concerns for most of us. There are some general rules one can follow for prevention of cardiovascular disease through nutrition.

Rule One: Reduce the intake of red meat. In a society

largely composed of "meat and potatoes" eaters, this may be a little hard to take, but the evidence shows that a massively animal-protein-laden diet is not of great benefit to anyone except athletes and others who regularly undergo great exertion. Unless a middle-aged, pot-bellied executive finds some way to burn off the excess energy he is taking in from his red-meat-dominated eating habits, he is simply giving his body more animal fat and protein than it can handle. Fatty build-ups are a reasonable expectation from a life of consumption of large amounts of meat.

We are not suggesting a wholesale abandonment of beef and beef products, unless the reader is already under therapy for a specific condition. The idea is to *reduce* the amount of red meat and to eat lean meats in place of fat-laden meats when possible. Fish and poultry are good substitutes for some of the red meat dishes.

Rule Two: Reduce the amount of milk and dairy products. These are animal fats and proteins and, except in cases of protein deficiency, are not necessary in anywhere near the amounts normally consumed in the United States. Milk itself is not necessary for adults and, if taken at all, is probably better for us in its raw (unpasteurized), skim, or lowfat varieties. Once again, the complete elimination of these products is not necessary; we are merely advocating a reduction in their consumption.

Rule Three: More fruits and vegetables and their juices should be eaten. We need greater amounts of fresh, naturally grown, and raw fruits and vegetables for their natural nutrients. They should be as fresh as possible, and raw or cooked as little as possible, because the longer they are stored and the more they are tampered with, preserved, frozen and/or cooked, the more they lose their natural vitamins and minerals. Seeds and kernels of fruits and vegetables should also be consumed.

A juicer or blender is useful for creating natural fruit and vegetable juices.

Rule Four: Eliminate or markedly reduce the amount of refined carbohydrates. Those people who have any form of glucose metabolism dysfunction should completely eliminate refined carbohydrates in their many forms. As a preventive measure, no one should consume more than a very limited quantity of refined carbohydrates.

111

Rule Five: Reduce the amount of stimulants consumed. There are few habits as deadly as the morning cups of coffee accompanied by several cigarettes. The noxious effects of cigarette smoking have become more and more obvious.

The addiction of Americans to caffeine is damaging to health and occurs in several forms. The most common addiction is to coffee, but tea, except for most herb teas, also contains caffeine. Cola drinks are especially damaging to the body because of their high sugar content and their caffeine.

Rule Six: Avoid all preservatives and artificially colored foods as much as possible. Not only are foods produced with these less nutritious, but some of the preservatives, dyes, and other chemicals are inferentially linked to cancer.

Rule Seven: Avoid contamination with vaporized chemicals and heavy metals. When they are unavoidable at work, home, or office, wear a mask. If you smoke, stop if possible. If you cannot stop smoking, then switch to a pipe, in which the heat, tar, and other contaminates are concentrated in the bowl.

Rule Eight: Have regular examinations by your doctor, and if even remote symptoms occur have noninvasive vascular studies performed. Insist on a properly performed six-hour glucose tolerance test if you score 20 or more on the Health Indicator Test. Have a hair analysis for trace mineral nutrients and toxic metals at least yearly, and where indicated, take specific trace mineral nutrients.

In addition to these eight rules, vitamins A, B complex, and C should be taken, and adequate exercise should take place daily. If these are all incorporated into a lifestyle without excessive stress, a person will have gone a long way toward prolonging his life and avoiding the heart disease catastrophe of the modern era.

FOUR

Cancer: Public Enemy Number Two

DISMAL FAILURE

The National Center for Health Statistics, which keeps track of such things, announced that in 1976 the overall death rate in this country declined for the first time in history. Even the number of deaths caused by heart disease had decreased. There were only three mortality-rate categories that increased between 1973 and 1975 as compared to the previous two-year period: cancer (the only "natural" killer on the list), murder, and suicide.

The 4.2 percent increase in fatalities from cancer was something of a shock to the field marshals of the so-called War on Cancer, the combined public-private initiative to wipe out cancer launched during the Nixon era. More than $5 billion in public and private research monies had been spent on that war by 1977, but by then, even the cautiously optimistic earlier assessments of the over-all cancer picture were giving way to gloom and doom.

The figures speak for themselves. In 1976, according to the official tally, at least 380,000 Americans died from cancer, and the actual figure was probably closer to 400,000 since many deaths due to the treatment of cancer are not officially ascribed to cancer in the statistics.

It is now estimated that throughout 1977 about 1,100 Americans were dying per day of cancer and that one out of every four Americans will eventually develop cancer. It has been projected that 54 million Americans now living will be hit by the disease.

Cancer is now pandemic, trailing only that combination of conditions called heart disease as the major natural killer. In the 1970s it is the leading killer of children and is rapidly becoming the number one killer of middle-aged women.

But these rates, however awesome for the United States, trail those for Great Britain. A general pattern has become obvious: the major industrial nations of western and northern Europe, North America, Australia, New Zealand, and Japan are areas in which cancer is rapidly gaining on heart disease as the most lethal of the Killer Diseases. But in the "emerging" countries, infections and parasitic diseases as well as basic malnutrition continue to be the major concerns, and cancer rates are nowhere near the level attained by the more "civilized" countries.

Heart disease still ranks as the number one killer in America, but it is cancer that is most feared. In a recent Gallup poll, 58 percent said that the condition they most feared was cancer, while only 10 percent chose heart disease. Perhaps this is because there are so many people walking around who are suffering from, yet somehow surviving, a "heart condition." The same can hardly be said for cancer. When it has metastasized, or spread, from one tissue to another there is little chance of surviving five months, let alone five years. In spite of the publicity drives of the American Cancer Society, the public relations staff of the Food and Drug Administration, and local medical societies, cancer means death for two out of every three victims, either from the disease itself or from the treatment of the disease.

There are those who say that cancer rates have not increased as much as it may seem, since the rates would have been higher in earlier years if cancer had always been properly diagnosed and not mistaken for other diseases in many cases. While there is probably some truth in this statement, it does not make the current figures any better. The statistical evidence is still overwhelming that never before have the number of cases or the fatalities from cancer been so high. President Ford's Council on Environmental Quality said as much in early 1976 when it reported that, although there had been twice as many cases of cancer since 1900, there had been

114

virtually no improvement in cancer survival rates since the 1950s.

This is the statistical background against which the current War on Cancer propaganda must be borne in mind. Optimistic news about "new breakthroughs" and "more favorable results" from orthodox therapy have little meaning when arrayed against these gruesome figures.

Tragically, research on cancer in the United States and much of the Western world continues to be focused almost exclusively on the hunt for human cancer–causing viruses and the production of new and more potent chemotherapeutic agents—that is, poisons—to kill cancer cells. The treatments of choice for cancer remain poisoning (chemotherapy), burning (radiation), and cutting (surgery).

Despite statistical juggling by medical orthodoxy in a seemingly continual effort not to rock the boat and to continue doing the same ineffectual things, these approaches have not reduced the incidence of cancer, and with the exception of a few varieties of cancer and some cancers detected sufficiently early, they have had no measurable overall effect in "curing" cancer. In fact, these methods have even been suspected in helping to spread the disease.

Such time-honored orthodox detection methods and treatments of cancer as mammography (breast X-rays) and estrogen came under sharp attack in 1976: American cancer authorities were told that the mammography program might cause 15 cases of cancer while saving the lives through early detection of only 5 of every 100,000 women under 50 years old.

And the female hormone estrogen, frequently used as a cancer *treatment* in both men and women, came under suspicion because of a combined Harvard School of Public Health and National Cancer Institute study in which estrogen was found to be a possible *cause* of breast cancer, thus challenging a 35-year-old medical tradition. About the same time, an article in the *Journal of the American Medical Association* warned that women routinely treated with estrogen are running the risk of developing uterine cancer at about the same rate as pack-a-day smokers risk lung cancer.

University of California physiologist Hardin Jones reported

that 23 years of cancer data convinced him that, statistically, a cancer patient will live longer and feel better if he or she opts to do nothing at all about the cancer rather than submit to chemotherapy and radiation, both of which so pulverize the body's immune system that, whether the cancer is affected or not, any minor infection may kill the patient.

In addition, the 66th Annual Meeting of the American Association for Cancer Research was told in 1976 that several drugs that have been used in the successful treatment of various forms of cancer may be responsible for the development of secondary tumors. Such common anticancer drugs as vincristine, nitrogen mustard, chlorambucil, procarbazine, phenylalanine mustard (L-PAM), and prednisone have all come under suspicion.

At the time of this writing, some 40 orthodox chemotherapeutic agents, all poisons of varying degrees of toxicity, are "drugs of choice," along with radiation and selective surgery, in grappling with the cancer pandemic. But do these therapies or combinations of them work?

The minimal increase in survival rates since the 1950s is probably due, more than anything else, to antibiotics and improved blood transfusion and operation techniques. Researcher Daniel Greenberg, publisher of *Science and Government Newsletter,* published an analysis of the War on Cancer by anonymous spokesmen at cancer institutes throughout the country. These people privately admitted that the War on Cancer was no closer to being won than the war in Southeast Asia had been, despite the mellifluous reports of "an end in sight" and "new breakthroughs expected" emanating from Washington.

The conclusion reached by Greenberg was that the slight improvement in cancer recovery rates since the 1950s is due not to more patients surviving cancer but to their survival of operations for cancer, operations that in an earlier era would have killed them.

Indeed, except for some scattered but promising work in anticancer vaccines and more attention being given to the manipulation of the body's natural defense mechanism or immune system, there was very little in the way of authentic optimism on the horizon for cancer treatment. Billions of dollars of tax and private monies continued to be poured into the development of new cytotoxins and/or their combinations and

116

the relentless pursuit of viruses thought to induce cancer in humans.

With the exception of skin cancer, uterine and cervical cancer in women, Hodgkin's disease, and childhood leukemia (the last two accounting for only about 2 percent of all cancer), it was still appropriate in the mid-1970s to assess the statistics relayed by former National Cancer Institute Director Frank Rauscher, Jr., to mean that a cancer victim using orthodox modalities of treatment had little more than a 7.5 percent chance to survive for five years. Meetings of cancer specialists, and their own in-house medical materials, consistently turned up litanies of failure through chemotherapy, radiation, and selective surgery, even when the very modest numbers of healthy survivors of this carnage were pointed to as proof positive of orthodoxy's triumph against the mass killer.

The War on Cancer, declared in 1971 and operational in 1972, had its first five-year assessment in congressional hearings in the summer of 1977. During these first accountings of the effort to pump billions of dollars into the hunt for the causes and cures of cancer, the entire program took a shellacking from several experts in the field. They told Representative L. H. Fountain's Government Operations Committee that the War on Cancer was mismanaged and nearly worthless, that viruses do not cause most human cancer, that the hunt for a cancer vaccine had been a "fiasco," and that the cancer-cure rate had not improved since 1957.

Dr. Howard Temin, a Nobel Prize–winning cancer virologist from the University of Wisconsin, testified:

> We can now say that infectious viruses like those that cause many human diseases do not cause most human cancer. Therefore, we cannot hope to develop a vaccine against a virus to prevent most human cancer. . . . We do not now have the fundamental knowledge to prevent or cure most human cancer.

"We do not now have the fundamental knowledge to prevent or cure most human cancer." This statement should reverberate down orthodoxy's hallowed halls.

Dr. Irwin Bross of Roswell Park Memorial Institute for Cancer Research in Buffalo, New York, told the legislators that much of the money Congress had earmarked for the cancer program had been "wasted on scientific boondoggles such as the worthless cancer vaccine program" and that the programs to detect environmental cancer-causers amounted to "little more than public relations gimmicks—paper tigers to reassure the concerned public that something is being done when it isn't."

He added, "This is standard policy in the NIH [National Institutes of Health]. The program on cigarette health hazards is a farce. It consists of noisy scare campaigns which are counter-productive—like most of cancer education."

Dr. Bross labelled the National Cancer Institute's efforts to develop a cancer vaccine "a fiasco—a waste of time, effort and hundreds of millions of taxpayers' dollars. If even half these [vaccine] resources had been put into an effective primary prevention program, we would at this moment be well on our way to the actual conquest of cancer."

Dr. Sidney M. Wolfe, a health consultant to Ralph Nader's consumer crusaders, told the Fountain committee, "Prevention cuts into the profit margin of existing industries, which have thus far been able to escape the costs of the cancer they cause. NCI, under new leadership, must choose to become the leader in the war to prevent cancer rather than the banking operation for the largely unsuccessful war to treat it after it happens."

At the same time, American cancer orthodoxy plays fast and loose with the word *cure*. As it is used, *cure* refers to *five years* of freedom from cancer's *symptoms*, usually tumors. That many people experience a return of cancer's symptoms six—or even 10 or more—years later does little to undercut orthodoxy's preoccupation with the five-year "cure" rate.

To even the most monolithically minded oncological surgeon who might take the time to read new data, it was becoming apparent in this decade that cancer, the rapidly fulminating scourge of the civilized world, must surely somehow be linked to factors in man's natural environment. Even while a cancer specialist might still be in the horrible position of defending the failure of orthodoxy in cancer treatment, he still need not have felt, as this decade opened, that he was being too unorthodox by looking at the wholesale evidence that cancer is, as an earlier researcher pointed out, almost entirely a *disease of civilization.*

The evidence is abundant: the connection between lung cancer and smoking, the linkage of specific varieties of cancer to certain industries and to certain materials (such as asbestos and vinyl chloride), the revelations that the widely used coloring agent "Red Dye No. 2" was at least statistically bound to various kinds of cancer in laboratory animals, the unresolved but suspicious connection between food additives and dyes and potential cancer, the inferential links between our lead-laced polluted air over urban areas and lung cancer, and the shocking and controversial studies by National Health Federation researchers which in 1974–75 statistically connected fluoridated water with higher cancer rates in fluoridated areas.

Evidence is mounting that additives, coloring agents, and unnatural chemicals of all kinds, added to the food supply of the civilized world to enhance, enrich, color, preserve, and entice, may be connected somehow with the induction of cancer —information absolutely unwelcome to the food processing industry, which, as we have seen, is a major culprit, even if unintentionally, in this nation's galloping descent into degenerative disease. Dr. Jacqueline Verrett, a veteran researcher with the Food and Drug Administration, has taken up the cudgels against such food industry items as the hormone diethylstilbestrol (DES), employed for the rapid fattening of cattle, and sodium nitrate and sodium nitrite, used to give meat a red color and to prevent botulism, all of which, she pointed out, may directly or indirectly be cancer-causing agents. She and others have argued that food processors have pressured the FDA to allow such possible inducers of human cancer to remain on the market while tests continue.

We have stressed that for a cell to remain healthy, it must receive the right nutrients at the right time and in the right proportions with other nutrients. In the increasingly abnormal environment of civilized man, with an industrially polluted air supply, a contaminated water supply, and the continual ingestion of denaturalized processed foods, multiple factors are well under way to sabotage the correct provision of nutrients to cells. Perhaps the only miracle here is that more cells do not go awry earlier among more people. But evolution has indeed produced a tough human species that is surviving, if agonizingly, the wholesale assault on its biological reality by the synthetic world of civilization.

In fact, there are clues now of thousands of possible *inducers* of cancer in civilized man, including, ironically enough, some of the orthodox drugs given to treat the tumors thereby produced. But only recently has attention begun—grudgingly, in the camp of orthodoxy—to be given not so much to the *cause* of cancer, but to its *prevention*. Indeed, prevention seems to be a word that strikes fear into the heart of that combination of disciplines, vested interests, and basic theories that comprise the core and marrow of the health-care delivery industry, approximately 80 percent of which is targeted for the treatment of degenerative disease.

Greenberg found in analyzing the losing War on Cancer that the most novel, if indeed suppressed, idea among American cancer researchers by 1975 was prevention. It simply made schoolboy sense: If treatment is a manifest failure, then why not look at what seems to prevent, or may prevent, cancer? The quiet voices in the American cancer establishment were joined by louder voices from without—for example, Dr. Alexander Pavlov, assistant director of the World Health Organization, who noted that it is easier to prevent cancer than to treat it, and that the discovery of a "cure" for cancer is still decades away.

Prevention of cancer, just as prevention of degenerative disease across the board, is a nettlesome, upsetting notion to the "club," that coalition of vested interests, highly paid surgeons and radiologists, and purveyors of expensive toxic drugs and special equipment involved in cancer treatment—to say nothing of the food processors who uncomfortably feel the degenerative-disease finger of suspicion pointing at them. Neither medical orthodoxy, nor the drug cartel, nor the food processing industry has a vested financial interest in probing deeply into cancer prevention. Nevertheless, they do have a human stake in it, of course, since cancer afflicts these ladies and gentlemen with the same savagery as the rest of the civilized population.

But in terms of long-range human stake versus short-term vested interest, it is frequent that the latter wins out—not because those involved in what we may call the "Cancer Establishment" are venal, but because they are human.

The nation's cancer bill for 1976 was conservatively set at about $25 *billion*—a figure comprehensible only in terms of astronomy. That figure includes an estimate of man-hours lost due to cancer, but a general compilation of the costs of (and thus profits accruing to the treatment of) cancer by 1976 indicates an amount somewhere between $15 and $20 *billion*. Included are costly hospital rooms, medical insurance, cancer surgery, cancer drugs, cancer-connected anesthesia, cancer-connected internal medicine, diagnosis, and follow-ups. It is not uncommon for "terminal" cancer patients to spend up to $50,000 from the onset of the initial "palpable mass" to entombment. Treatment is awesomely expensive, and the salaries of cancer specialists are sky-high.

The cost of treating Americans for cancer (and the figures here refer to *direct* costs, not indirect or hidden ones) was estimated for 1976 at 4 to 5 percent of the nation's total health bill, or about $5 billion. The 1974 assessment of the nation's total health bill was about $100 billion, but indirect costs and inflation set it as high as $140 billion by 1976, of which up to $20 billion, including direct and indirect (hidden) costs, could safely be attributed to cancer. The estimate in 1976 was that 1.3 million Americans are hospitalized for cancer each year, with an average hospital stay of at least 26 days. One single element of the "cancer industry" can be seen from these figures alone: assuming that hospital rooms cost, conservatively, $100 a day, $338 million is spent each year for the cost of rooms alone, without any medication, surgery, or other treatment.

Cancer has become both the celebrity disease and the most feared of the degenerative Killers, in spite of the fact that it is heart disease, not cancer, that is responsible for more than half the deaths each year.

As Dr. Bergman says in *The Solid Gold Stethoscope*, "Cancer has pizzazz, box office, and glamour, and in actual dollars and prestige, even heart and mental [disease] can't hold a candle to it. It's a health dodge with a future and everybody who's anybody is jumping in, especially politicians. (Who votes against a cure for cancer?)"

The American Cancer Society (ACS) was established in 1913 on an "emergency" basis. It has now become a huge, largely ineffective organization that spends less on research than on employee salaries, benefits, and "education."

In the fiscal year ending August 31, 1975, the last year for which figures are currently available, the ACS received $109.8 million in donations and $12.1 million from investments, for a total of $121.9 million. Of this, $59 million went to such things as travel, salaries, office rent for close to 3,000 offices, office supplies, and publications. Another $21 million was put in reserve to bring the total unspent assets of the organization to a reported $155 million.

Most of the generous American public that donates the massive funds assumes that the lion's share of the money collected will be used to directly fight cancer through assisting cancer victims and/or research to conquer the disease. But this simply is not true. Only $5.7 million went to direct aid to cancer victims, and only $31.2 million went for research during the same time that the organization collected a total of $121.9 million. And very little of the money that was spent on research went very far afield from the rigid—and losing—parameters on medical "orthodoxy."

It is no wonder that all the fund-drive hoopla of the ACS and the enormous infusion of research money by the federal government have not been able to dent either the incidence of cancer or the fatality statistics. Neither the public sector nor the private one, usually represented by the ACS, seemed willing to spend a bit of their funds on unorthodoxy other than the first timid steps taken at the federal level, and against the agonizing wails of the old guard, into the dietary aspects of cancer.

As this is written, it is safe to say that, despite the horrendous reality that almost 1,100 Americans are dying daily of cancer, more people are living *off* the disease than dying *from* it!

The results of orthodoxy statistically are extremely bad, as we have seen. However, the human effects are even worse. Cancer is one of those diseases, we are told by the medically orthodox, in which the patient is supposed to feel worse in order to get better. As thousands of barely surviving victims of chemotherapy and radiation will admit, their treatments are frequently worse than death itself. The horrible sequelae of burned, charred skin, literally cooked internal organs, the falling out of hair, the persistent fatigue and malaise and hours of intense nausea are the side-effects of chemotherapy and radiation in a majority of cases. Some of the drugs are so poisonous that they have known fatality levels in and of themselves.

The thinking behind this treatment approach is almost medieval: if cancer is construed as a disease characterized by palpable tumefactions—"lump and bump disease"—then the full force of the "most modern treatment" is brought to bear in cutting off, blasting out, burning, or poisoning the lumps and bumps. The body is invaded by immune system–destroying poisons that are supposed to kill cancer cells before these same agents kill the body.

It is quite true that radiation and chemotherapy are very frequently able to reduce the size of tumors—but the ringer here is that tumors characteristically are composed of up to 90 percent normal, or somatic, tissue and represent the body's natural efforts at self-healing by surrounding the malignancy with malignancy-mimicking and natural encapsulation. To the extent that tumors are reduced by burning and poisoning, the body's natural tissues have been attacked and badly damaged. The surgical excision of a single tumor *may* end the cancer crisis, unless the mere act of cutting, as sometimes happens, itself spreads the cancer.

To a growing body of the allegedly unorthodox—the metabolic therapists—cancer is not lump and bump disease at all. Lumps and bumps are, indeed, *symptoms* of what these therapists see as a systemic, chronic, *metabolic* disease. To these physicians, the overwhelming preoccupation of orthodoxy with cutting off tumors or poisoning and burning them—save in those directly life-threatening situations (say, a tumor on the windpipe) in which immediate heroic efforts must be used —is akin to medical orthodoxy's view in Renaissance times that treatment of the skin lesions of both syphilis and small-pox (the "great" and "lesser" pox) was the equivalent of treating the diseases themselves.

What if cancer *is* a systemic, chronic, metabolic disease of which lumps and bumps constitute only symptoms? Will this not mean that billions of dollars have been misspent and that the basic premises on which cancer treatment and research are grounded are wrong? Of course it will, and in decades to come a perplexed future generation will look back in amazement on how current medicine approached cancer with the cobalt machine, the surgical knife, and the introduction of poisons into the system and wonder if such brutality really occurred.

As the failure of orthodoxy in cancer becomes more abundantly clear, and as hundreds of thousands of cancer patients, brutalized beyond belief through the techniques of cut-burn-and-poison, grasp at that last final straw, the "miracle cure" offered by everything from prayer and medication to herbal treatments and seaweed, the honest minds of the medical establishment are beginning to look into unorthodoxy—and to prevention. They are being forced by basic human logic and the sheer failure of the War on Cancer to look at the one open road that cuts through the confusion over both cancer prevention and treatment. That one open road is *nutrition.*

THE DIETARY LINK

Until 1975–76, to have an interest in and to seek information about links between nutrition and cancer was regarded as latter-day quackery. With a medical establishment composed of virologists, radiologists, surgeons, and developers and purveyors of toxic poisons for cancer management, the concept that foods somehow play a role in preventing, inducing, or managing cancer constituted viscerally unwelcome information.

But a few team players kept plugging away anyway, among them Dr. Ernst L. Wynder, president of the American Health Foundation, New York, who for several years has made the appropriate link between diet and cancer, and who even went so far as to suggest that the "prudent diet" advanced as a means of preventing heart disease might also be useful in heading off cancer. Basically, the prudent diet involves reducing fat intake, reducing cholesterol to 300 milligrams per day, and eating no more than four eggs per week and red meat no more than four times per week. As we shall see, this prudent anticardiovascular disease diet is remarkably parallel, in a major sense, to the prevention and treatment diet advanced by the exponents of metabolic therapy in cancer. (Our suggestions on diet are presented in chapter five.)

Dr. Wynder early noticed that Japanese who adjust to American dietary habits (and who thus may be easily compared with homeland Japanese remaining on the basic Japanese diet) develop American cholesterol levels, acquire American rates of heart disease, and get the same levels and kinds of cancer. He and other researchers have also noted that upper-income groups in Japan are acquiring colon and breast cancer at levels which seem to overlap their adoption of Western diets. In the matter of breast cancer, the suspicion that diet is implicated was voiced by the World Health Organization in 1975, when a WHO report naming this kind of malignancy the major killer of women between 35 and 54 noted that breast cancer rates are far higher in western and northern Europe and North America than elsewhere in the world and that "specialists are studying a theory that something in the Oriental diet provides a form of protection" against the disease.

Earlier, a study of Seventh-Day Adventists in the United States, including those who inhabit this nation's most atmospherically polluted area, the Los Angeles basin, sparked some genuine interest in nutrition because of the demonstration of lower rates of colon, pancreas, breast, and prostate cancers for members of this religious sect when compared to the population at large.

Since the basic age, sex, and racial percentages of Adventists are the same as the surrounding population, and since they are exposed to the same contaminants in their basic lives, then what is the primary variable in their habits that relates to dramatically lower incidences of cancer?

The Adventists are essentially, but not totally, vegetarians, and consume less meat in general than the surrounding population. Also, they generally abstain from smoking and drinking. But their generally lower levels of cancer cannot be ascribed only to less smoking and drinking. Clearly the dietary variable is of extreme importance.

More than a year after the Adventist study appeared, the *New England Journal of Medicine* came up with another puzzler that has even deeper ramifications: the much lower incidence of cancer among white residents of Utah as compared with the American population at large was ascribed to the fact that 72 percent of Utahans are Mormons and that Mormons, among other things, generally do not consume alcohol and tobacco.

But again, this proscription could hardly account for the overall lower incidence of cancers of the stomach, liver and kidney among men, and of the breast and uterine cervix among women, and the lower rates in general of colonic, rectal, and pancreatic cancer. Here, vegetarianism itself could not be a key issue since the Mormons are not, in general, a vegetarian population, even though dietary moderation does seem to be general among them.

In early 1976, Dr. Robert A. Good, president and director of research at the Memorial Sloan-Kettering Cancer Center, told Fairchild News Service that immunotherapy—the triggering of the body's natural defense system to fight disease—holds great promise in combating cancer. He added that while no one yet knows all the determining factors that cause the immune system to react to a given agent, he and his colleagues had, in his words, "stumbled across one interesting idea—nutrition—as a means of manipulating the immune system." Indeed, he added, "we have found that we could increase or decrease immunity efficiency by varying the nutritional content of the diet—in fact we have doubled the life expectancy of a certain strain of mice through nutritional manipulation."

The idea that Good and his colleagues had "stumbled across" was, of course, not new at all—though the orthodox elite at Sloan-Kettering, Roswell Park and other prestigious Establishment cancer centers may think so. The concept of preventive diet in cancer is one of the major cornerstones of what the Establishment has heretofore called quackery.

As early as the 1930s, the highly respected physician, Dr. Max Gerson, was pioneering the connection between nutrition and cancer, and in terms of treatment he advanced case after case to prove that a radical change in diet, accompanied by a vigorous "detoxification" program, constituted the answer to cancer. For all his pioneering efforts, Dr. Gerson—later called by Albert Schweitzer "a medical genius who walked among us"—was damned as a nutritional quack and declared a fraud by the New York County Medical Society.

Naturopaths, "health food cranks," homeopaths, and a handful of medical doctors had talked and written about diet and nutrition in cancer and indeed in all disease for years, but these individuals were essentially written off as outside-the-pale eccentrics not to be taken seriously.

But with WHO and such club members as Dr. Good beginning to note the cancer-nutrition link by the mid-1970s, this area of "quackery" was gaining an iota of legitimacy. Immunotherapy itself had been seen as little more than sophisticated quackery a decade before.

By 1976, four Nobel Prize winners could testify that 50 percent or more of cancer is due to nutritional deficiencies, and five scientists were able to tell Congress that Americans who failed to eat a balanced diet or who eat too much are promoting their chances for cancer. But the same scientists were cautious when asked for details on what specific foods and brands would be either good or bad for an individual.

Dr. Gio B. Gori, deputy director of the National Cancer Institute's division of cancer cause and prevention, told the Senate Select Nutrition Committee that improper diets are related to 60 percent of all types of cancer in women and 41 percent of those in men.

His testimony, and that of others in 1976, tended to focus on excessive intake of meat, sugars, starches, and fats, including those fats in meat.

In what the metabolic physicians regarded as a breakthrough in the Establishment point of view regarding cancer, Nicholas Gonzalez wrote in such a lay-oriented but Establishment-okayed journal as *Family Health/Today's Health* that diet seems to be the major variable among certain populations studied for cancer rates, and that peoples who shift geographic locales and are exposed to the dietary habits of the new host nations take on the cancer rates of the host populations—a datum which, if borne out by further research, would even make nutritional aspects of cancer perhaps more important than a possible genetic inclination to the disease. The Gonzalez article, entitled "Preventing," reflected a point of view that, just a few years before, had been regarded as utterly ridiculous by the medical establishment of the United States and much of the Western world.

It is a half-skip from linking nutrition and cancer to examining the various nutrients involved—namely, vitamins— and this mini-step opens up a whole new area of thought and concern in the cancer war. It brings in the entire area of metabolic therapy, holistic medicine and outright disease prevention through supplying the right amounts of the right nutrients at the right time so that cells can continue to flourish in optimum health.

Vitamins in therapy, let alone prevention, have been even less welcome to American medical orthodoxy than the idea of nutrition, and the harshest attacks of Establishment power have been reserved for the orthomolecular therapists who stress megadoses of vitamins as essential to the management of disease. But while the U.S. has looked askance at vitamins, Europe has forged ahead on several fronts.

A Swiss research center and a Vanderbilt University team in the United States have reported dramatic evidence that treatment with vitamin A reverses the effects of cancer. The same researchers have pointed out that nearly one in every three Americans suffers from some degree of vitamin A deficiency, which itself may leave them dangerously vulnerable to cancer-causing substances.

Vanderbilt's Dr. Frank Chytill said: "With Vitamin A therapy, doctors now have a way to restore body cells to normal—rather than destroy them with surgery, chemotherapy, or radiation. We now have laboratory evidence that cancers such as breast, lung and skin tumors can be cured by treatment with Vitamin A." His coresearcher, Dr. David Ong, noted: "We know that lack of Vitamin A retards normal growth, weakens the mucous linings of the body, and causes night blindness. But when the proper level of Vitamin A is restored, the body returns to normal. Work with patients in Europe strongly indicates that Vitamin A works the same way with cancer."

At the famed Janker Radiation Clinic in Bonn, West Germany, writer Patrick M. McGrady found the Germans doing some relatively spectacular cancer research with vitamin A–emulsion therapy, but he was not holding his breath in expectation that American medical officialdom would be too interested.

"Poor America"—he wrote in an *Esquire* article entitled "The American Cancer Society Means Well but the Janker Clinic Means Better"—"Its money-fat, guts-thin biomedical research establishment has more and more to do with paper and abstract mathematics and fear and less and less to do with new therapies or even with people suffering from cancer. If it would only send some good doctors to the Janker Clinic, it might not only learn something about cancer care, but it might get a good lesson or two in freedom."

The Janker Clinic is also the producer of Wobe-Mugos proteolytic (protein-digesting) enzymes, substances indirectly banned from use in the United States along with the outlawed Laetrile therapy. These enzymes are used either as adjuvant treatment along with Laetrile, other vitamins, minerals, and enzymes, or as a treatment in their own right, since information is rapidly gathering on their ability to strip cancer cells of their protective "shield," thus allowing the body's immune system to attack and destroy the cells.

The tendency of the American medical establishment not to follow up on such seemingly unwanted disciplines as megavitamin therapy is even more scandalous as it relates to vitamin C. The published literature on aspects of vitamin C, or ascorbic acid, as it relates to cancer is actually extensive, yet few American doctors are knowledgeable on the subject. But chemist and researcher Irwin Stone, two-time Nobel Prize winner Linus Pauling, and Dr. Ewan Cameron have kept the subject before the public and have done important, indeed vital, research on vitamin C and malignancy.

Stone, arguing that man's inability to produce ascorbate brings on a lifelong condition that he terms "chronic subclinical scurvy," a precursor state to the full range of degenerative disease, has researched and written extensively on the use of huge doses of ascorbate of vitamin C in the treatment of cancer, including such evidence as total remission of myelogenous leukemia with up to 42 grams of vitamin C daily.

In 1969, Dean Burk, Ph.D., cytochemistry chief of the National Cancer Institute—and vociferous backer of Laetrile, or vitamin B_{17}, from within the very bowels of the Establishment—showed in a paper published in *Oncology* that ascorbate kills cancer cells while doing no harm to normal cells. Burk and his group indicated that vitamin C doses as high as the equivalent of *three quarters of a pound* in a 150-pound man were administered to animals without "notable pharmacological effects."

They wrote: "In our view, the future of effective cancer chemotherapy will not rest on the use of host-toxic compounds now so widely employed, but upon virtually host non-toxic compounds that are lethal to cancer cells of which ascorbate ... represents an excellent prototype." They also discovered that vitamin C had never been tested for anticancer effects by

129

the Cancer Chemotherapy National Service Center, because it was too *non*toxic to fit into their screening programs! Analyzed Irwin Stone:

> They [orthodoxy] don't want to test anything unless it helps kill the cancer patient.
>
> A substance like ascorbate that will kill cancer cells and be harmless to normal cells has been a long-term goal and dream of cancer researchers, and in 1969 it looked like it had been achieved. One would expect that a crash research program would immediately be organized to thoroughly check and extend these observations and obtain clinical data on this breakthrough. That was seven years ago and no further papers could be found that were published by the National Cancer Institute on this important subject.

By 1976, the National Cancer Institute had an $800 million budget, with less than $6 million of it going into nutrition research, and even this amount was fought by old-line bureaucrats but was forced on them by congressional mandate, according to columnist Jack Anderson.

The result of bureaucratic foot-dragging on the cancer-nutrition front, Anderson recorded, is that the United States is now trailing England, Scotland, and the Soviet Union in important aspects of such research. At the same time, Dr. Pauling was finding it impossible to get federal funds for his vitamin C–cancer research, and both Dr. Jorgen Schlegel, who had made significant progress in fighting cancer with vitamin A at Tulane Medical School, and Dr. Eli Seifter, who was the first to demonstrate that vitamin A could be used against tumors of probable viral origin, were refused funds to further their work.

But in April, 1977, it was announced that a timid step would be taken by orthodoxy to check out the possibilities of vitamin A—in its less-toxic, synthetic form—against cancer.

In what represents a significant breakthrough at the National Cancer Institute, so long committed to the defense of radiation and the hunt for new toxic chemotherapeutic agents in the losing War on Cancer, it was announced that a nationwide study of a drug "related" to vitamin A would be undertaken at nine research institutions to see if its use could *prevent* bladder cancer.

The drug in question is 13-cis-retinoic acid, a synthetic vitamin A belonging to a family of compounds called "retinoids," a term that NCI spokesmen emphasized in an effort to de-emphasize the outright association with vitamin A.

The vitamin A–type chemicals were selected for study because of the accruing evidence that they play key roles in the growth and repair processes of the epithelial cells that cover the external and internal surfaces of the body. These surface cells—found in the lungs, stomach, uterus, intestines, kidney, prostate, testes, pancreas, and skin—are involved in more than half of all human cancer.

It should be stressed here that the vitamin A and C research bears more on treating an existing condition rather than preventing it. It should also be pointed out that the timid steps by American medical orthodoxy into the previously never-never land of diet are by no means indicative of anything like general opinion. It still remains an open question as to what kinds of diet might be implied in the cancer incidence variables, and the debate over the amount of fiber in the diet and the role of fats, sugars, and starches is far from over.

The dietary elements of cancer are in two areas: the degree to which pollutants and additives in foods, and the denaturalization of foods themselves, may actually induce, or play a role in inducing, cancer; and the degree to which diet alone—the amounts, excesses, or lack of nutrients—is involved.

The bridge between the allegedly quack world of the metabolic, nutrition-oriented therapists and the adherents of the viral theory of cancer and the cut-burn-and-poison school of tumorcide may have already been supplied by the immunologists, who note that the body's immune system is the first line of defense against *all* disease, and who are now increasingly realizing that diet plays a key role in the immune system.

The chief elements in the immune system attack on cancer are the assault on malignant cells by lymphocytes or white-blood cells, and, secondarily, the apparent role of pancreatic enzymes in the same attack. But the degree to which the immune system is suppressed or weakened by cancer is an unsolved problem. In the malnourished the first line of defense may be weak, or virtually nonexistent. Some favorable results have been achieved by the administration of "transfer factor," an immunological molecule (polypeptide) from the bloodstream of a donor to the bloodstream of a patient. This "trans-

131

ferred" immunity aids host lymphocytes in the attack on cancer.

But of even more importance is the examination of two other elements:

First, just how do the multiple poisons that surround civilized man actually induce cancer—that is, how do they cause a normal cell to become a wildly proliferating one? Or do they really do this directly at all?

Second, to what extent do dietary habits influence the immune system? How can whole groups of humans subjected to the same poisons and toxic chemicals as the rest of us, be statistically cancer-free or at least exhibit far lower rates of cancer?

It is ironic, if not shocking, that following an expenditure of $5 billion in the War on Cancer, and with a $120 million per year budget available from the American Cancer Society, it is still not known precisely *if* or *which* alleged viruses cause cancer in man and just how a normal cell becomes an "abnormal" one—or even if this is actually the cancer-induction process itself. The fact that *in vitro* laboratory studies associate certain kinds of viruses with tumors does not mean that the viruses caused the tumors; it is almost as appropriate to say that cancers cause viruses as it is to state that viruses cause cancer, yet the "theory of choice" in Western oncology by the mid-1970s has remained that viruses somehow cause a malignant transformation.

There is the growing, and exciting, possibility that cancer may *not* be the 100-plus separate diseases with 100-plus allied similar demonstrations it is now thought to be, but that it is a single disease, in which malnutrition, polluting poisons, and the like—all due to the physiological and mental stresses of civilization—play a role as causers of cancer. The damaged tissue resulting from the malnutrition and poisons then become more susceptible to attack by viruses, bacteria, and parasites.

In fact, in the raging controversy over vitamin B_{17}, or Laetrile, the evidence is rapidly accumulating that cancer is, more than anything else, a specific vitamin-deficiency disease, and that the best approach to its treatment is in total metabolic therapy, or holistic medicine, through dietary manipulation and the administration of enzymes, vitamins, and minerals. More important, evidence is also mounting that even in a civilized world of toxic chemicals, pollutants, and atmospheric poisons, the restoration of a vital food factor to the denaturalized diet of the Western world may very well be the answer to cancer—and that cancer may be eliminated as surely in one generation as a killer disease as pellagra, scurvy, pernicious anemia and other vitamin deficiency diseases were in earlier eras.

LAETRILE (VITAMIN B17)

When, in 1971, a Kansas salesman named Glen Rutherford was diagnosed as having invasive adenocarcinoma of the lower intestine—bowel cancer—he was told that immediate surgery was necessary and that he might have to lose his rectum.

This disquieting information, following a long siege of intestinal complaints and bleeding and accompanied by discovery of an orange-sized tumor, sent the independent-minded Rutherford smack into the arms of unorthodoxy—that is, he made the trip, as so many Americans have, to Tijuana, Mexico, to a clinic specializing in the use of vitamin B17, or Laetrile, in cancer therapy.

Rutherford's case is of double interest because, although the diagnosis was made in the United States by a "legitimate" clinic, he eschewed all orthodox treatment to seek the novel approach being done, legally and openly, in Mexico, one of more than two dozen countries where the use of Laetrile, indirectly outlawed in the United States through Food and Drug Administration regulations on interstate shipment and sale, is either legal for use or otherwise not interfered with by government bureaucracy.

Under Dr. Carlos Lopez at the Centro Medico Del Mar clinic in Tijuana, Rutherford was placed on several weeks of "Laetrile therapy"—a radical alteration of his diet in which all animal protein was barred (milk, eggs, red meat, dairy products), and in which raw, fresh fruits and vegetables and their juices were substituted. Along with this, he was given protein-digesting enzymes, a battery of vitamins, and, most particularly, intravenous injections of Laetrile.

The first response to the treatment, Rutherford recalls, was cessation of the rectal bleeding he had been undergoing for several months. Within the same few weeks' period, the orange-sized tumor mass shrank to the size of a grape. At that time, clinic doctors cauterized it—the only orthodox modality used during his treatment, and one which anti-Laetrile voices in the United States would later refer to as the real reason for his control over cancer. The shrinking of the tumor from the size of an orange to the size of a grape has frequently been referred to as a "spontaneous remission." This is a favorite explanation of conventional oncologists when faced with a control or alleviation of cancer tissue by unorthodox, "unapproved" methods.

Rutherford returned to the United States, but had follow-up examinations thereafter. Sticking religiously to the anti-cancer eating plan, and gulping down vitamins and tablets of Laetrile every day, the Kansan remained free of all symptoms of cancer in his first year of treatment. By 1977, when he became the eye of a growing Laetrile hurricane, he had completed six years free of symptoms (a "cure" in normal cancer parlance). Not that he considers himself "cured"—"controlled" is the favored adjective used by metabolic therapists to describe completely positive response to a regimen of vitamins including large amounts of vitamin B_{17}, enzymes, and dietary manipulation.

Rutherford, like so many "controllees," went on to become a vocal exponent of Laetrile. He was the first in a growing number of patients listed as plaintiffs in a class action suit against the U.S. government that won the right of "terminal" cancer patients to be able to receive supplies of foreign Laetrile by court order without interference by the FDA.

The federal class-action suit of 1975 was only one of a series of maneuvers that brought the controversy over Laetrile and the murkiness of the laws involved into full swing.

Laetrile proponents estimated that as of 1977 at least 75,000 Americans and Canadians were using, or had been using, Laetrile either for cancer prevention or treatment, despite their governments' long-time disavowals of the substance as a quack remedy. While unavailable as a product for a quarter-century before, Laetrile, a nontoxic substance, had been the most hounded of the unorthodox cancer remedies, but unlike such unwanted putative cancer fighters as Dr. William Koch's glyoxylide, Dr. Andrew Ivy's Krebiozen, and the Harry Hoxsey herbal treatments from the same era in which Laetrile was developed, Laetrile—backed by a political and lobbying effort—was fighting back.

By the mid-1970s, the American Cancer Society had termed Laetrile the "number-one problem in cancer quackery" and, in combination with the FDA and local medical societies, was conducting a heated campaign against it. The arrests of vitamin distributors, entrapments of Laetrile suppliers, and the blanket indictment of 16 people—and conviction of four—in a so-called international Laetrile smuggling ring helped bring matters to a head. As apricot kernels—a rich natural source of Laetrile—were confiscated by the ton in raids across the nation, and as the plight of physicians and pharmacists arrested or harassed for their use or distribution of Laetrile became known, the outcry of the American people began to be heard. By mid-1977, as the "Laetrile War" raged white-hot, a Louis Harris Poll showed that 54 percent of Americans believed that cancer patients should have the right to have Laetrile, whether orthodoxy agreed with it or not, and 63 percent believed state legislatures had the right to circumvent the FDA's unwritten ban on interstate shipment and sale of the taboo material. Yet the voices of orthodoxy continued to write off Laetrile as a worthless nostrum and a hoax on the public.

But despite the clamors of American orthodoxy, some substantial information about the research on Laetrile has been forthcoming from a number of sources. The Laetrile-using clinics in Mexico, one of them in operation for 15 years, by 1977 were reporting "positive response" rates on cancer in about 65 to 68 percent of cases, a figure doubly remarkable when it is realized that of these patients some 95 percent, mostly Americans, had already been judged terminal, and most of them had suffered through the effects of chemotherapy, radiation, and/or surgery with no real relief. Most of those responding were on the full metabolic program of B_{17} diet, vitamins, and enzymes, but some others were showing improvement with the use of Laetrile along with standard therapies.

135

The recovery of Alycia Buttons, wife of the American comedian Red Buttons, and of another person who is the wife of a noted cosmetics entrepreneur, by the use of Laetrile, brought the name of Dr. Hans Nieper of West Germany to the forefront. Nieper had been using large doses of Laetrile, sometimes mixed with zinc orotate as "activated amygdalin," for some time, and drawing clients from the United States and Europe. Indeed, West Germany was fast becoming a center for modified Laetrile treatment and production.

In the Philippines, Dr. Manuel D. Navarro, at the Santo Tomás University Hospital research center, continued intriguing work that linked the low cancer incidence in the Philippines with natural sources of vitamin B_{17}, and also reported positive responses to Laetrile and allied treatment on almost a thousand patients whose records he had kept during two decades.

An Israeli medical team, investigating the Tijuana clinics and several U.S. doctors who use metabolic therapy based on vitamin B_{17}, reported favorably on the substance, and Israel began using the compound in 1976. A number of clinics throughout the world are using Laetrile as an ancillary therapy or as the basis of a total metabolic program while this is being written, despite continuing damnation of "the worthless apricot-pit cancer cure" by the American cancer establishment.

At this writing, Laetrile is "legal" for cancer therapy in 27 countries—though "legal" does not mean in any case approved as a "drug of choice." In several countries, such as Australia, Laetrile may be used by a physician by special permission although its distribution is illegal. In many other countries, its use is simply not interfered with because government agencies are not responsible for controlling medications *per se*. Laetrile attained statutory legality in Mexico and may be freely shipped for private use to most countries. In several countries, the use of Laetrile is "cleared" for experimental use but its general distribution is not allowed. Its use is still marginal, but growing, and Mexican factories provide the great majority of both the injectable and tablet forms of Laetrile used in North America. Factories in West Germany and Monte Carlo also produce considerable amounts of the product.

Also at this writing, California was the only state with specific anti-Laetrile laws on the books, but those were being challenged as California became one of almost 40 states in which active legislation to decriminalize the use of Laetrile was underway in 1977. The pressure on medics *not* to use Laetrile was not only statutory—as in California—but indirect, as in most states, where physicians who use "unproven remedies" may be punished by their state boards of medical examiners. In some states, "cancer advisory commissions" are allowed to pass on the legitimacy of medication used in cancer management. The right of such boards to make such judgments, and of government to intervene in any way in the doctor-patient relationship, was at the root of the "freedom-of-choice" controversy that was sweeping America as this book went to press.

The Committee for Freedom of Choice in Cancer Therapy, Inc., the primary pro-Laetrile lobbying group, was set up in 1972 to defend a California physician hauled into court on "cancer quackery" charges for using vitamin B_{17}. The committee estimates that no more than five doctors in the country *openly* used Laetrile in 1972, but by 1977 that number had risen to more than 60—of about 1,200 who were using or providing it "on the sly" and who were members of the rapidly growing organization.

While only a handful of these doctors were metabolic therapists in the full sense of the term, even these few were providing dramatic new information on the therapeutic uses of vitamin B_{17} along with a total program of dietary change, vitamins, enzymes, and minerals.

E. Paul Wedel, M.D., of Salem, Oregon, himself a Laetrile-controlled cancer patient, reported that half of about 5,000 cancer patients he had treated with total metabolic therapy over several years were doing "reasonably well" and that more than 200 had undergone "total remission," or seeming total control, of their cancers, most of which had been regarded as terminal.

Philip E. Binzel, M.D., of Washington Court House, Ohio, reported in 1976 that his experience with two-and-a-half years of B_{17}-based metabolic therapy on cancer patients showed that 88 percent were still alive, 77 percent could be described as "well," and some 33 percent indicated the cancer had been stopped or controlled.

John A. Richardson, M.D., of Albany, California, around

137

whose 1972 arrest swirled the court cases and allied politics that converted Laetrile into the "freedom of choice" movement, reported by 1976 that well over 60 percent of about 6,000 patients he had treated had shown "positive response" to B_{17}-based metabolic treatment. The positive responses ranged from cessation of cancer-connected pain and subjective feelings of well-being to stimulated appetite, weight gain, blocking of metastasis and, in some cases, total remission of all symptoms. Richardson's license to practice medicine was revoked in late 1976.

James Privitera, M.D., West Covina, California, among the California doctors arrested on Laetrile-connected charges, stated in court affidavits that "at least 70 percent of all my patients who have cancer have experienced very substantial or dramatic improvement in all of the four categories of improvement [increase in well-being, increase in appetite, gain in weight and decrease of pain], and up to 90 percent of all such patients improve to some extent, at least, or even substantially, in one or more of such categories of improvement."

Even more dramatic results were forthcoming the same year from Tijuana's Dr. Ernesto Contreras, perhaps the most experienced Laetrile therapist in the field, and the man to whose staff up to 60,000 Americans had turned for some kind of cancer relief in his clinic's 14 years of operation. In a report prepared for the Mexican government—which had legalized the use of Laetrile under its chemical term in Spanish (*amigdalina,* for amygdalin) as an analgesic in lung cancer—Dr. Contreras reported some 67 percent "positive responses" among the 5,000 best-documented sets of records he was monitoring. This is an incredible score for a cluster of cancer patients almost all of whom had been given up as hopeless by American orthodoxy.

Among the more astounding of the Contreras records were three cases of persons who survived for five years after having inoperable lung cancer, including two from deadly oatcell carcinoma, a variety of lung tumor that the Americans are reluctant to even treat through orthodox methods. All made their five-year survivals—the period of time orthodoxy usually requires before claiming a cancer "cure"—on Laetrile and its ancillary therapy.

Dr. Contreras and his staff were also finding, as did the staff at the new Cydel Clinic in Tijuana, that relatively large doses of nontoxic Laetrile (9 to 12 grams intravenously) could be mixed with low levels of the orthodox toxic chemicals to provide at least sudden and dramatic tumor reduction, with the metabolically fascinating discovery that patients so treated no longer suffered the harmful side effects of such standard poisonous agents as 5-fluorouracil (5-FU) and cyclophosphamide.

Throughout the United States, as Laetrile evidence grew, an increasing number of cases appeared along the lines of that of Glen Rutherford—individuals treated *only* with Laetrile and its total program and who had rejected, or not been subjected to, chemotherapy, radiation, and selective surgery. The case of Pam McDaniel, referred to earlier in this book, was among them.

The metabolic therapists reporting on the use of Laetrile and its total metabolic program are thus reporting a success rate far in excess of the successes achieved through standard, orthodox treatment. But success must not only be thought of in terms of "hanging on to the last thread of life." Even more important is the quality of life, and if a metabolic program including vitamin B_{17} can relieve the pain and suffering of hopeless victims of the disease for their remaining life, then it becomes a valuable asset in the medical armamentarium.

The medical records mentioned, and the thousands of new testimonial case histories by Americans either treated abroad or somewhat sub rosa in their own country were routinely referred to by the cancer establishment and medical orthodoxy as "anecdotal" or as "spontaneous remissions."

Worse, government forces even sought to bar popular access to the raw material from which most Laetrile used in North America is manufactured—apricot kernels—by referring to the fact that the vitamin B_{17} within (amygdalin) contains a cyanide radical, and stressing the toxicity of cyanide. Metabolic therapists and Laetrile adherents shot back that the refined product is absolutely nontoxic (or at least less toxic than aspirin) at doses as high as 70 grams intravenous per day, and that, save from allergenic reactions by some people, the consumption of the raw, natural vitamin B_{17} in the form of apricot kernels is also harmless unless *biologically unreasonable amounts* are consumed in unsound ways that might enhance the possibility of a cyanide release (more of the seeds than would be present in the amount of fruit that one would normally consume at any one time).

As the Laetrile controversy erupted fully on both scientific and political fronts, orthodoxy essentially admitted that the apricot kernel extract itself was harmless, and argued primarily that since it was "worthless," its danger to the public lay in diverting time and energy away from a cancer patient's access to orthodox modalities—the achievement record for which, as we have seen, renders such an argument hollow.

In addition, if a person wishes to undertake both types of treatment at once, this is, of course, possible. The only reason we do not advocate the use of chemotoxic agents and radiation is that they may do damage that cannot be reversed by the body's defense mechanism or by Vitamin B_{17}. However, in studies by Dr. Mario Soto in Mexico City and at Tijuana's Cydel Clinic in which chemotoxic agents and Laetrile or radiation and Laetrile have been used together, success rates have been superior to those cases in which Laetrile did not accompany these types of treatments. In addition, the side effects of nausea, loss of hair, cachexia, et cetera, that often accompany chemotoxic agents and radiation were absent or greatly reduced when Laetrile was used.

The incredible lengths to which entrenched Establishment and the positive animal test results using Laetrile may be inferred from two scandals in Laetrile's turbulent quarter-century history in the United States.

Even though the vitamin nature of Laetrile was postulated in 1970, and the growing thought of the advocates of Laetrile was that a vitamin itself could not be "legal" or "illegal," an effort to legally license Laetrile in accordance with Food, Drug and Cosmetic Act guidelines, and at considerable expense, was made in 1970 by the McNaughton Foundation, then conducting Laetrile research in the United States and Canada. This followed two earlier, less exhaustive efforts.

It should be pointed out that the reasons now given by Laetrile advocates for not seeking licensing of Laetrile are that (1) vitamin B_{17}, a food, is neither a drug nor a food additive, and thus does not fall under those categories controlled by the FDA, and (2) since there is no meaningful patent on the substance itself, there is no way to recover the estimated $10 to $15 million expenditure that would be involved in licensing a medical substance through the current FDA machinery,

140

a process that could take anywhere from five to ten years.

But in 1970 the McNaughton Foundation decided to go ahead with efforts to secure the full official blessing of the controversial substance anyway. In late April, 1970, the FDA issued an "investigational new drug order," or IND, to the McNaughton Foundation which would have allowed the foundation to initiate clinical (human) studies of amygdalin. The IND was issued based on a mountain of information submitted by the foundation, which detailed the substance's success in its early clinical uses in the 1950s and scattered if impressive animal research data since then.

Then, less than two weeks later, the go-ahead was suddenly revoked, allegedly at the behest of a key official who had testified in anti-Laetrile cases in the 1950s. The excuse given was that "serious pre-clinical deficiencies" in the McNaughton Foundation submission were found. The organization was given ten days to "correct the deficiencies" and to cease clinical studies. Significantly enough, the foundation *did* comply with the sending of additional information, which went into the mail within the allotted time, but the FDA claimed that the foundation had failed to adhere to its orders, so the short-lived IND was terminated in May, 1970.

The only thing such action accomplished was the reinforcement of the alleged paranoia of the Laetrile promoters and the enhancing of their distrust of the governmental bureaucracy, which they see as the policing wing of vested interests threatened by the vitamin theory of cancer and the potentially inexpensive treatment that would be posed by producing synthetic Laetrile from any of its hundreds of natural sources.

Equally scandalous, if not more so, was the ongoing suppression, at Memorial Sloan-Kettering Cancer Center in New York, of positive results of amygdalin in experiments on mice especially bred to develop spontaneous mammary cancer.

In the period 1973–75, at least six sets of raw data from tests conducted by Dr. Kanematsu Sugiura, a veteran research scientist, were "leaked" by individuals at the center. The tests showed that amygdalin effectively blocked the spread of cancer in the test animals and had some effect in inhibiting tumors. Laetrile (amygdalin) was also associated with apparent increases in the animals' longevity and improved health. These tests, of course, invalidate the claims of

141

orthodoxy that Laetrile "has never passed animal tests" and that neither a "valid sign of efficacy" nor a "shred of evidence" has ever been detected in animal trials or human use that would justify beginning full scale clinical tests.

Through a stormy era (1975–77) in which Sloan-Kettering spokesmen issued various contradictory statements and, abetted by major news media, sought to create the impression that an initial Sugiura test had been a "fluke," outside journalists began to sense that there was more to the tests than met the eye. A national news syndicate reported that early results of a "double blind" test used to check out Sugiura's results (since a number of other experimenters had, according to Sloan-Kettering, been unable to "replicate" the scientist's findings) had been at least partially positive. Then, in the fall of 1976, it was learned that the double blind study had been aborted because a number of the test mice had been accidentally killed.

At this point a group of Sloan-Kettering employees issued its own report, claiming that positive Laetrile results had, in fact, been covered up, including the most recent double blind study, which had turned out to be "positive." Moreover, added the employee group in its own in-house publication: "The record shows that the top leaders of SKI are terrified of reporting ANY positive results with Laetrile, even if these are modified by more negative findings. The issue is no longer whether or not Laetrile works, but the political and economic embarrassment these men and their colleagues will feel if Laetrile turns out to have even a shred of value."

They added,

Laetrile is relatively cheap, plentiful, non-toxic and non-patentable. It is, however, everything an anti-cancer drug should *not* be, from the point of view of the drug companies and the medical bureaucrats. [The latter] have their own reasons for opposing this substance. Twenty-five years ago some prominent California doctors performed a study of cancer patients treated with a weak solution of the substance, and found it ineffective. Since that time, doctor has dogmatically followed doctor in condemning it, according to the unwritten code of the "medical fraternity." In fact, most of the leaders of the "war on cancer" are now on record damning Laetrile. They no more relish being proven wrong than their counterparts in the Vietnam War did ten years ago.

The new Sloan-Kettering disclosures meant that *at least* seven sets of animal studies had indicated at least *some* efficacy with Laetrile—and that efficacy resulted even with Laetrile given alone, not as a metabolic agent along with a total nutritional program that has been shown to give even better results. Even more ironic is the fact that virtually *no* chemotherapeutic agent has been found effective against the variety of cancer being studied. In addition, *no* studies have ever indicated that Laetrile might produce cancer in test animals, unlike a number of the orthodox and legal modalities, which *are* associated with cancer in laboratory animals and even in humans.

In summer 1977, Sloan-Kettering again attempted to end the controversy by announcing an abstract of results of all the Laetrile tests on mice over several years. In so doing, SKI spokesmen made much of the failure of Laetrile in *transplanted* tumors, admitted that Dr. Sugiura had achieved some results with *spontaneous* tumors (and that a Sugiura co-worker had at least partial success in one test), but argued that since no other scientist had been able to "replicate" Sugiura's results completely the institute's position was still that Laetrile was worthless in cancer treatment.

But even as SKI was attempting to unload its hottest potato since one of its researchers had been caught doctoring results of experiments in mice in an earlier, non-Laetrile-related scandal, work by independent investigators on animal models was tending to confirm Sugiura's results. Biologist Harold W. Manner at Loyola University, Chicago, was proving in a carefully constructed series of experiments (1) the nontoxicity of Laetrile at even irrationally high doses and (2) its ability— and that of other vitamins—to help prevent cancer. In September 1977 he announced the total regression of tumors in 84 test mice with mammary cancer using a daily regimen of Laetrile, vitamin A, and proteolytic enzymes. At Salisbury State College, Salisbury, Maryland, biologist Vern van Breemen was indicating with a two-year investigation an almost 100 percent blockage of the development of spontaneous mammary cancer in mice simply by adding apricot kernels to their normal diet.

As the question of efficacy of Laetrile as it pertains to *animal* experiments—none of these in any way fulfilling the protocols of a *total metabolic therapy*—remained murky, orthodoxy by mid-1977 desperately shifted its emphasis to the supposed "danger" of natural vitamin B17 and the single case of a baby's death due to putative cyanide poisoning after she *may* have consumed one or more Laetrile tablets. While to scientific observers such an argument remained ludicrous—inasmuch as the 40 "legal" anticancer drugs are known to be poisonous and such over-the-counter medicines as aspirin result in many poisonings and toxic reactions per year—there was a certain shock effect on the public. But at a hearing before the Senate Health Subcommittee in Washington, during which the massed forces of orthodoxy attempted once and for all to discredit Laetrile, veteran cancer researcher and biotoxicologist Bruce Halstead, M.D., with a single presentation virtually demolished the argument of Laetrile toxicity. The hearing had been called as the wave of states rushing to decriminalize Laetrile grew and as major media efforts to stop Laetrile through ad hominem attacks on its promoters began to fail.

At the hearing, it was brought out that one recent test showed that the experimental animal toxicity range for Laetrile is 3,000 milligrams per kilogram of body weight—or the equivalent of 210 *grams* for a 154-pound man! Such facts seemed to matter little, as long as the word *cyanide* was present to scare the uninitiated. Orthodoxy in 1976 and 1977 produced reports indicating that populations that rely heavily on B17-compound-containing diets may experience a number of physiological complaints believed to be linked to cyanide poisoning. Such surveys were efforts to discredit Laetrile and avoided the central argument that *natural* vitamin B17–containing foods may bear the "unlocking" enzyme for the B17 compound as well as the B17 compound itself, thus increasing the chances for toxicity, while Laetrile is a refined product *without* the "unlocking" enzyme. Also brought to attention were scattered cases in which some cancer patients were suffering from short-term side effects of Laetrile use—but these effects, metabolic therapists pointed out, are due to the body's inability to detoxify itself fast enough following the rapid destruction of cancer cells. In other words, some of these rarely reported effects simply indicate that Laetrile is *working*.

Not content with attacks on Laetrile for its "cyanide radical" content and the scattered cases of allergenic, noncyanide side effects, the new FDA commissioner announced a "serious public health hazard" from Laetrile because of alleged instances of "microbial contamination" and "adulteration." These "disclosures" followed seizure by federal agents of large shipments of Mexican Laetrile, a raid on the only Laetrile tablet manufacturer in the United States, and one-by-one examination of seized tablets and vials of the substance. Laetrile proponents responded that such cases of contamination and adulteration constituted arguments *for* decriminalization, legalization, standardization, and quality control of *American* Laetrile. They also pointed out that, nothwithstanding the FDA's declarations, at least 75,000 Americans and Canadians were using Laetrile daily without any negative effects.

But these governmental allegations and blendings of fact and fancy served to bolster the new attack on Laetrile: No longer was it worthless though harmless. Now it was worthless and potentially harmful. Laetrile proponents saw in such tactics a grasp-at-any-straw effort to use every conceivable measure to stamp out the existence and growing use of a refined product that, by any rational measure, remained for all intents and purposes utterly nontoxic at even megadose levels.

Thus the scientific controversy over Laetrile became as political as a war, and that controversy continues to rage as testimonials to its benefits pour in, only to be routinely dismissed by the Establishment as "purely anecdotal" or "hearsay."

There were exciting, if difficult to document, cases in which patients claimed a definite metastasis-blocking or tumor-inhibiting effect simply from heavy ingestion of apricot kernels and such vitamin B_{17}–containing foods as peach kernels. And two California veterinarians reported anticancer effects in domesticated cats and dogs from use of either vitamin B_{17} in the natural state or in the refined Laetrile form.

It is interesting to note that domesticated cats and dogs have a very high incidence of cancer and heart disease, while those living in the wild, independent of man's selection of contaminated food, polluted water, and toxic air, have never been known to suffer from these major killers. The wild animals' biological selectivity of food sources, when untampered with by man, maintains a high immunological response and resistance to the degenerative Killer Diseases (cancer and heart disease).

While the controversy around Laetrile focused primarily on cancer *treatment,* and whether patients and doctors did or did not have the right to a nontoxic alternative cancer therapy with the Laetrile program (a point won in favor of Laetrile when Alaska, as of September 21, 1976, allowed the legal use of Laetrile therapy in that state; 12 states had followed suit by mid-1977), the pioneers of the Laetrile movement were suggesting that the far more exciting element in the controversy is the *preventive* aspect of vitamin B_{17}.

It has been Dr. Harper's position for many years that primary responsibility for the inception of the original cell that later develops into "lumps and bumps" lies with at least two factors: (1) malnutrition—that is, the inadequate delivery of the proper nutrients in the proper amounts at the proper time to the proper location, and in the proper combination, and (2) specific toxins that, singly or in combination, interfere with the cellular metabolism of normal cells, with the result that, at the time of subdivision, progressively more abnormal cells are produced that malfunction as the deficiency continues and the toxicity of the cell increases.

The malfunction of the cells that make up the organ systems is therefore responsible for the primary effects (symptoms) of aging. At some point during mitosis (cell division), the RNA-DNA molecule of the nucleus becomes disarranged and results in cells of abnormal growth patterns. As this progression continues, the cells become more and more abnormal until the original first predecessor (one individual cell) creates lumps and bumps through wild proliferation.

This position has also been advanced in statements made by many researchers, including recent Nobel Prize winners, who have stated that more than 50 percent of cancer cases in the United States are the result of malnutrition and that additionally the pollution of air, water, and food is paramount in the causation of cancer.

Ernst T. Krebs, Jr., the embattled San Francisco biochemist who with his late father, a medical doctor, named and developed Laetrile, has advanced the theory that cancer is not only linked to diet and nutrition but that it is, indeed, a specific vitamin-deficiency disease, the deficiency being in the class of chemicals variously known as cyanophoric glucosides, beta-cyanogenetic glucosides, or nitrilosides, and which Krebs baptized vitamin B_{17} because of their nontoxic and water-soluble nature and their virtual ubiquity in the plant kingdom.

The vitamin theory of cancer, and the specific classification of amygdalin and amygdalinlike compounds as vitamin B_{17}, was not expostulated until 1969, well after Laetrile's introduction as an antineoplastic agent in 1950—which, in turn, was well after the introduction of a crude form of the extract in the 1920s. Krebs' position is that cancer is the result of unchecked trophoblast cells (see below) running wild because the first line of defense against them, the immune system and pancreatic enzymes, are inefficient or not working, and also because the second line of defense, natural vitamin B_{17}, is not present in the diet.

After discussions and debates between Dr. Harper and the Laetrile champions, the latter reconsidered the possibility of causative factors or organizers of cancer tissue other than solely vitamin B_{17} deficiency, and many of them would agree that there are several *causes* of cancer.

Krebs stunned audiences around the country as he proclaimed that sufficient ingestion of vitamin B_{17} in a myriad of its natural forms (but most positively through consumption of the seeds of apricots and peaches, which contain up to 3 percent pure amygdalin) would be a virtual guarantee of a life free from clinical cancer despite exposure of the body to the full range of chemicals, poisons, pollutants and associated tissue-attackers so abundant in the civilized world.

Moreover, Krebs has argued that vitamin B_{17} fully conforms to a vitamin classification—a point disputed by orthodoxy—by providing a wide range of metabolic effects, among them a reduction in hypertension and probable positive effects against the hemolytic crisis of sickle-cell anemia.

Krebs has insisted his focus is the outright *prevention* of cancer through natural ingestion of vitamin B_{17}, a substance inadvertently removed from "civilized" diets by social customs (for example, spitting out fruit seeds instead of eating them), economics (substituting wheat for millet, a natural source of B_{17}), and food processing, which has stripped so many natural nutrients out of the food consumed in industrialized countries.

A mighty combination of vested interests and orthodox belief was not pleased with the theory that cancer—like scurvy or pellagra—might be a simple vitamin-deficiency disease, and Laetrile received the same suppressive treatment that had earlier been given to Max Gerson's views, as well as to the agents glyoxylide, Krebiozen, and the herbal remedies.

But the Laetrile movement would not die, and at some point in the late 1960s it began to merge with the overlapping interest in health foods, vegetarianism, vitamins, and ortho-molecular therapy to become the total therapeutic package it is now—one which is showing such dramatically beneficial results and an achievement level so superior to orthodoxy that its major activists and advocates are the thousands of people on the program and their relatives, friends, and loved ones.

The claims made for Laetrile treatment are, after all, modest—in distinction to what the American Cancer Society, the FDA, and other institutions claim that the Laetrile adherents are saying about vitamin B_{17}.

With the hindsight of historic experience in the B_{17} dietary management program behind us, we can make the following assertions:

The Laetrile program cannot restore lost or damaged tissue. That is, patients who have already been devastated either by cancer or by treatment for cancer based on radiation, chemotherapy, and surgery cannot hope for the restoration of tissue, nor can they count on surviving cancer or the effects of their earlier treatment for cancer. It is no "miracle cure."

The most recurring direct response to Laetrile injections is relief from cancer-connected pain, a single element that is a blessing in and of itself for many thousands of cancer sufferers and their families. In many cases of terminal cancer, this is the only noticeable response, but an important one, for it usually means the patient no longer needs addictive opiates.

The majority of Laetrile-program-treated patients reports favorable responses in terms of increased appetite and weight gain and developing a more cheerful outlook. Cancer is awesomely depressing, and with its demonstrable induction of loss of appetite—many cancer patients actually die from cachexia, or slow starvation—it produces mentally reinforcing periods of pessimism. The Laetrile program seems to cut this cycle and often very quickly.

In many cases, the complete elimination of cancer-connected fetor (stench) is also reported.

In summation, most persons on the Laetrile-treatment program simply start *feeling better*. This does not mean they will miraculously recover either from cancer or from the extreme damage done to them by the disease and/or by earlier treatment. This is one reason why most Laetrile advocates point out that the earlier a person turns to the total treatment program, and the more completely he has avoided standard orthodox therapy alone, the better he is apt to fare under Laetrile management.

Since Western medicine still essentially regards cancer as a lump and bump disease, patients and clinicians new to Laetrile are frequently obsessed with whether or not tumors are being directly affected by the treatment.

Topical use of Laetrile has in fact been associated with rapid and dramatic effects on tumors, but we stress again that since cancer is an underlying, systemic, chronic, metabolic disease, appearances of tumors are only symptoms, and they are signs not only of cancer but how the body is *responding*— or even *if* it is responding—to cancer. That's why, under the early Laetrile regimen, there may actually be an *increase* in tumors. But such increase actually means the body's immune system is being stimulated to do battle *against* cancer, for, again, the majority of a tumor is natural—not cancerous—tissue, and the bigger the lump or bump is, the more filled it is with natural (somatic) tissue. The absence of tumors does not mean there is not still subclinical malignancy, nor does the existence of tumors mean that cancer has not been checked. In many cases, the Laetrile program continues while tumors stay in the same numbers and sizes until they are "benign." They may then be surgically excised or left alone. They may even simply disappear.

In many cases simple surgical excision of the tumor tissue may be indicated either before, during, or after the implementation of a total metabolic program. However, by itself, surgical excision of the lump or bump does not correct the underlying metabolic deficiency or metabolic toxicity, nor does it activate the body's immunological response to fight the abnormal cells.

The fallacy of surgical intervention alone in the treatment of cancer is well demonstrated when there is a wide excision of the tumor such as in a radical mastectomy, which involves the removal of the breast and the excision of underlying muscles and the lymph nodes under the arm. There is commonly a recurrence of cancer tissue (lumps or bumps) along the surgical incision, or a different kind of cancer may begin in an entirely new location.

149

Both animal studies and human case histories have abundantly indicated that primary tumors or malignancies, unless they immediately threaten life (as, for example, those on the windpipe), are not the killers. What kills is the spread, or metastasis, of cancer from a primary site to other tissues. It has also been well demonstrated that the essential element of the Laetrile program is blocking the metastasis of cancer rather than its assault on a primary tumor. Theoretically, Laetrile as a single agent is far more effective on a developing, subclinical malignancy, and less effective on a tumor mass, and more effective on a tumor mass that is well situated near a blood supply, and less effective on tumors in bones or areas of difficult circulatory access. The probable subclinical destruction of malignant cells by Laetrile forms the bedrock theory for the natural prophylaxis or the outright prevention of cancer by both the "first team"—the body's immune system and the totality of the pancreatic enzymes indirectly killing off cancer cells almost as fast as they appear—and the "second team"— the cyanophoric glycosides whose unleashing of cyanide and benzaldehyde in one modus operandi or another provides a direct attack on the cells.

Patients recovering from cancer on the Laetrile program are routinely told to continue on vitamin B_{17} tablets and at least modified diets for the rest of their lives, for, theoretically, since the absence of vitamin B_{17} in the diet is seen as the single most important reason why cancer developed in the first place, then it is the inclusion of vitamin B_{17} in the diet that will effect continuing control of the disease. Some patients have reported control simply through abundant use of natural foods containing vitamin B_{17}, particularly apricot kernels and bitter almonds, but the maintenance level of tablets is suggested because they provide compact, highly refined large portions of amygdalin.

Laetrilists no more argue that Laetrile "cures" cancer any more than they would say insulin "cures" diabetes—but both substances may control their respective conditions.

Total metabolic treatment for cancer patients routinely consists of an immediate abandonment or severe limitation of animal protein, its substitution with raw, fresh, and/or sprouted vegetables, fruits, and unprocessed cereals, the administration of proteolytic enzymes, and usually vitamins A, C, and E,

150

as well as vitamin B15, or pangamic acid, the designation Krebs gave to another widely distributed food factor with an abundant range of metabolic effects. Along with this, minerals may be administered as needed, since many cases of cancer seem inextricably tied in with certain mineral deficiencies and almost certainly play a role in how the breakdown products of vitamin B17 are transported into cells.

The diet may be gradually relaxed according to individual cases, but patients seldom refer to themselves as "cured." This is in marked distinction to that minority of patients who survive orthodox treatment for cancer and are placed back in the same milieu, in terms of diet, from which they originally suffered cancer.

The Laetrile program has been effective against virtually every kind of cancer known, which does not surprise Laetrilists, for they consider cancer essentially to be one disease or condition with a multiplicity of forms and symptoms. The pandemicity of cancer in the industrialized nations, they believe, is far more due to the removal of vitamin B17 from the diet than it is to any other single factor—but the vast sea of carcinogens, or cancer-causing agents, in which civilized man exists, and the carcinogens in his processed foods and beverages and in the air he breathes, greatly exacerbate the B17-less condition so that, for all intents and purposes, the civilized man who has not already been attacked by another Killer Disease is only biding his time until clinically demonstrable cancer strikes.

THE NATURE AND INDUCTION OF CANCER

As of this writing, Western medical orthodoxy is in a quandary as to the actual induction of cancer, as we have seen, but even the more orthodox views of its cause are beginning to leave the door open to metabolic and/or megavitamin therapy in terms of treatment, and once the door is widely opened in terms of treatment, then dietary *prevention* of this Killer Disease is only inches away from recognition.

It is not fully understood how a so-called normal cell can be converted into a so-called malignant one—or even if this is the actual nature of cancer itself. But inasmuch as important links have been made between the occurrence of cancer and specific carcinogens, we should examine Western thinking about the onset of cancer, bearing in mind that oncology still regards cancer to be perhaps as many as 110 diseases, rather than—as the writers believe—probably *one* disease with many variables.

It has been noted that cell chemistry may be altered by changes of the cell membrane that may be spurred by specific carcinogens. The cell-chemistry alteration may be due to attack by the highly active molecular fragments called free radicals and one of whose effects may be the rancidification of cellular fats (lipid peroxidation).

In *Supernutrition,* biochemist Richard Passwater has strongly argued that the regulation of nutrients passing through altered membranes is itself altered and thus may lead either to the death of the normal cell or to its uncontrollable growth. The manner in which the latter is achieved has sparked a variety of theories, but primary among them are those that argue that a cell's genetic information (the DNA chain) may somehow become miscoded so that uncontrollable growth occurs.

This miscoding would be similar to the jamming of a computer—the computer being the genetically programmed DNA (deoxyribonucleic acid, the basic genetic molecule and protein producer and the single known substance that can reproduce itself). Because of a chemical transformation within the cell caused by alterations of the cell membrane (and these alterations are due to carcinogenic substances), the DNA program turns out to be different than the normal one. The new program is uncontrolled growth—malignancy—rather than the continued *suppression* of this growth.

But even if the various and interlocking theories on normal cell transformation to malignant growth are correct, the implication is growing that the "free-radical scavenger" vitamins such as vitamin E, substances that deactivate the free radicals, are vital in possible treatment and prevention.

Vitamins E and C and selenium are equally impressive as

possible protections against skin cancer, as are a host of substances that prevent oxidation (the antioxidants) in defense against cancer "caused" by radiation.

The comparatively recent interest in harnessing the body's immune system as the first line of defense against cancer—the production of antibodies and the whole overlapping series of chemical interchanges by which the body actually "treats" itself—has brought oncological orthodoxy ever closer to the vitamin B_{17}–related universe.

The bedrock theory of vitamin B_{17} as prevention and therapy in cancer, which stands as the most revolutionary approach to this seemingly complicated, misunderstood condition, is that the body's immune system, including the totality of the pancreatic enzymes, *is* the first line of defense against cancer and that, to the extent that this total system is not functioning, cancer may result, and that vitamin B_{17} constitutes the natural second line of defense—the "extrinsic factor" —in both prevention and control.

Moreover, advocates of Laetrile insist that the "scoop" about cancer is that cancer is a natural part of the lifecycle and that it is a condition caused by the *lack* of something, not *by* something. Adequate research has gone on in many countries including the United States, Canada, the Philippines and both Germanies, to bolster the Laetrilist position that pollutants in the air, water, and food, X-rays, overexposure to the sun, poisons from smoking, and the like are not causes but "organizers" of cancer. As we have pointed out earlier, it has been shown that there is an increased frequency of cancer of all types in a population exposed to lead pollution (11 percent cancer in 12 years) as compared with a population not exposed to this type of pollution (1.2 percent cancer in 12 years).

The advocates of this position take their cue from the late Scottish embryologist, John Beard (1857–1924), whose major contribution to embryology, and to cancer research, was his contention that the wildly proliferating cell that naturally arises in the life cycle to attack and eat out a niche in the uterine wall for the placement and nutrition of the embryo— the *trophoblast*—is one and the same as *cancer.* That is, the same development, outside the uterus, of trophoblast "at the wrong place and/or time" is *cancer.*

Beard noted the gradual development of the trophoblast from the primitive germ cell, the primordial cell of the lifecycle, and saw that since the trophoblast has a natural suppressing mechanism within the body, cancer must have the same suppressing mechanism. Subsequent "Beardians," as the men who continued his research have called themselves, have noted that without "natural cancer"—the trophoblast—life itself would be impossible. It is only when this natural cancer runs unchecked that it imperils the very life it has been essential in creating!

The Beardians have focused their attention on what it is that naturally suppresses the natural trophoblast. They learned, for example, that without the natural suppression of the trophoblast, the mother and the developing fetus would be dead of extremely malignant chorioepithelioma—cancer of the chorion—within a matter of days to weeks. Yet, almost always, something triggers the rapid destruction of the trophoblast once its single function in the lifecycle (attacking the uterine wall for the placement of the embryo) has been achieved, so chorioepithelioma almost never occurs.

They learned that it is the beginning of the functioning of the fetal pancreas that spells the death of the trophoblast cells at about the fifty-sixth day of pregnancy, and they have since focused on pancreatic enzymes, particularly chymotrypsin, as the destroyers of the trophoblast, not by direct attack as much as by the digestion of the electron coating surrounding the trophoblast, thus exposing it to direct attack by the body's immune system through the lymphocytes and probably exposing it to further digestion by the enzymes themselves.

Through the work of biochemist Ernst T. Krebs, Jr., co-pioneer of vitamins B_{15} and B_{17}, and other Beardians, research has continued from the 1940s to the present on Beardianism, but numerous problems remained. Among them:

Are *all* forms of cancer trophoblastic? And if they are, why shouldn't the single treatment for cancer be pancreatic enzymes? Exactly what is it that triggers a primitive germ cell into the eventual production of a trophoblast, or cancer?

Beard theorized that in the developing fetus a majority of primitive germ cells cluster in the gonads, there to await their eventual transformation into sperm or ova, but a minority of them—variously estimated from 20 to 30 percent—"migrate" at random through the body. These "leftover" germ cells could, under the appropriate conditions, transform not into sexually produced new entities, but *asexually* produced new entities—that is, cancer, "trophoblast at the wrong place and/or time." These leftover primitive germ cells might be found in any tissue, and only they could ultimately undergo the transformation into cancer.

Work by latter-day Beardians convinced them that the single triggering factor in the chain of events that causes a primitive germ cell to undergo differentiation ultimately into trophoblasts, or cancer, is the action of the female hormone estrogen. This point is still theory and not agreed upon by all Beardians, but if it is anywhere near the mark, it means that the "organizers" (X rays, overexposure to sunlight, et cetera) may, by causing a repeated abuse of the tissue—a damage to it—elicit estrogen for tissue repair. The contact of estrogen with a primitive germ cell sets off the chain reaction whose ultimate expression is trophoblast.

However, when the immune system is functioning adequately, as soon as cell differentiation to the point of trophoblast has occurred, the body's total immune system and the pancreatic enzymes are marshaled in immediate response to the "new, asexual pregnancy." The two Krebses and other Beardians have argued that a normal person has cancer many times during his lifetime, but the cancer may never reach the clinical stage because this natural intrinsic mechanism is operative.

Drs. Charles Gurchot, Franklin Shively, Krebs and others helped pioneer the use of chymotrypsin, a pancreatic enzyme, in cancer therapy, but with only mixed results. It was Dr. Gurchot, a pharmacologist and mentor of the younger Krebs, who recently updated the Beardian theory to explain how even a normal cell could, through chemical changes within it brought about by the alteration of its membrane by carcinogens, become a pretrophoblast cell, or primitive germ cell. His speculation is much in alignment with modern research on the possible effects of carcinogens in altering cell chemistry to the point at which "asexual generation" genes are abnormally activated. It closes the gap between considering cancer as possible *only* from the differentiation of the leftover primitive germ cells and considering that cancer may arise from *any* cell, particularly if that cell takes on the characteristics of a

155

primitive germ cell that will ultimately be expressed as trophoblast.

If the body responds to both the aberrant primitive germ cell and the aberrant natural, or somatic, cell whose asexual generation genes have been activated, then it becomes only a fine distinction to ponder whether the trophoblast, or cancer, is "natural" or "activated"—for as a rose is a rose is a rose, then a trophoblast, derived from either the aberrant germ cell or a somatic cell seemingly converted into, or mimicking, a primitive germ cell by the effects of carcinogenecity, still is, for all practical, biological purposes, cancer—and vice versa.

Ernst T. Krebs, Jr., turned his attention to looking for an *extrinsic* factor in cancer control, since the *intrinsic* one—the immune system and the totality of the pancreatic enzymes—remained insufficiently understood as the total answer. For that reason, he returned to the studies of the apricot kernel extract his father had earlier used, in conjunction with researchers around the world, in many successful treatments of cancer patients.*

Through trial and error, Krebs hit upon amygdalin, one of the better-known cyanophoric glycosides, as the probable active ingredient in the extract, and he pioneered the refined, crystallized, purified, and originally freeze-dried form of amygdalin for injection or tablet use as Laetrile—a name wrought from the chemical description *lae*vo-mandeloni*trile*. In so doing, Krebs had actually *returned* to the use of amygdalin in cancer therapy, for its first known modern-era application as a cancer fighter was reported as early as 1845, and there is also an insinuation that the ancient Chinese may have used a paste made from bitter almonds, a rich source of vitamin B17, on tumors thousands of years before Christ.

Intensive research by Krebs, backed by several other investigators abroad, increasingly convinced him that the whole

* It is not the province of this book to go into the fascinating story of Laetrile—the early research in the 1920s, the early use of the substance and its rejection by American medical orthodoxy, and the political and economic ramifications involved. The full story is told in *Vitamin B17: Forbidden Weapon Against Cancer* (New Rochelle, N.Y.: Arlington House, 1974) and *Freedom from Cancer* (Seal Beach, Calif.: '76 Press and Committee for Freedom of Choice in Cancer Therapy, Inc., 1976), both by Michael L. Culbert.

range of chemicals called cyanophoric glycosides or beta-cyanogenetic glucosides constitute, by the sum total of their metabolic effects, and their seeming specificity in cancer, a newly classified nontoxic, water-soluble, virtually ubiquitous B vitamin—vitamin B_{17}—and that its level in the diet constitutes the single most important element in the *prevention* of cancer and, very likely, one of the most important approaches in terms of cancer *treatment*.

Research has revealed that vitamin B_{17}, or any of the very similar beta-cyanogenetic chemicals of which amygdalin, prunasin, and linamarin are the most common, exists in some 1,400 plants, fruits, vegetables, grasses, and cereals, a ubiquity matched only by vitamin C. But, as Krebs *et al.* found, the modern "civilized" diet has almost completely removed vitamin B_{17} from ingestion by humans, due to food processing itself, which strips vitamin B_{17} along with many other things out of foods, and because of our eating customs—for example, the failure to consume seeds and kernels while opting for consumption of the fleshy meat of fruits. (Vitamin B_{17} is found in the seeds or kernels of virtually all fruits grown in North America except citrus fruits.) The change from millet to wheat for bread also removed an abundant source of the vitamin (which may also be found in buckwheat and barley groats).

In studying the worldwide epidemiology of cancer in relation to dietary intake, the Laetrile researchers have noted that specific populations studied for both (such as the primitive Eskimos of the Arctic, the Hunzakuts of northeast Pakistan, certain tribes in Nigeria, those Hopi and Navajo Indians in the United States who adhere to the diets of their forefathers, and, inferentially, the Vilcabamba Indians of Ecuador, the Abkhasians of the Soviet Union, and nonurban populations in Southeast Asia, particularly the rural Filipinos) have virtually nonexistent or vastly reduced rates of cancer—and, one might add, greatly reduced incidences of degenerative diseases across the board.

For two of these virtually cancer-free populations—the mostly carnivorous Arctic Eskimos and the mostly vegetarian Hunzakuts—the only major link is their apparently considerable ingestion of vitamin B_{17}, the Eskimos from the semidigested and highly nitrilosidic (vitamin B_{17}–bearing) tundra grass consumed by the caribou, on which the Eskimos have long fed, and the Hunzakuts from the continual ingestion of apricot kernels as snacks, and the consuming of nitrilosidic grains in their common bread. The recent studies of Seventh-Day Adventists in the United States also reflect a B17 component, since the selection of a mostly vegetarian diet will, by its very nature, restore considerable amounts of the vitamin to the diet.

The Philippines' Dr. Manuel D. Navarro in 1976 linked the low incidence of cancer in his native country (the incidence of cancer in Mindanao, for example, is a marginal one case per 100,000 inhabitants) to the extremely varied nitrilosidic diet of rural Filipinos, including the daily consumption of cassava and the frequent ingestion of a variety of B17-bearing beans, unpolished wild rice, and such delicacies as *papait,* the semi-digested grass from goat rumen, an Ilocano dish.

Krebs found in the almost universally abundant family of beta-cyanogenetic chemicals a new vitamin—one, he believes, that has been specifically selected by nature to be the "surveillant, anti-neoplastic vitamin," a harmless, nontoxic sentinel continually on duty to provide the *extrinsic* factor in cancer prevention, just as an adequately functioning immune system and the pancreatic enzymes together constitute the *intrinsic* first line of defense in cancer prevention. Using the axiom that "that which prevents also cures," Krebs elaborated the Laetrile theory of cancer treatment, since expanded to include a total metabolic program for the control of cancer.

Just how vitamin B17 "works" has been an important controversy almost since the beginning days of Laetrile research. The basic theory holds that cancer cells (or trophoblasts) are abundant in enzymes called *beta-glycosidases,* but deficient in the enzyme *rhodanese,* a known detoxifier of cyanide. The beta-glycosidases break the B17 compounds (usually amygdalin) into their component parts—glucose, cyanide, and benzaldehyde. The latter two selectively and synergistically attack the cancer, but do not attack natural rhodanese-protected tissue, converting instead to the harmless but useful chemical thiocyanate, normally excreted by the body.

This hypothesis has been called into question many times, and a number of elaborate theories as to how vitamin B17 works have been advanced. In the 1970s, evidence was mounting that cyanates, or metabolic breakdown products of cyanide-bearing compounds, surely inhibit cancer, but how to get them into the system and at what levels remained arguable. Additional interest is being given to the specific roles of other minerals and vitamins in conjunction with B_{17}, since the manner in which vitamin B_{17} is introduced into the body, the amount introduced, and the levels of specific minerals doubtless play essential roles in the delivery of B_{17}'s antineoplastic elements.

Intriguingly enough, while the voice of cancer orthodoxy has continued to claim that the Krebs chemical theory on the modus operandi of vitamin B_{17} has never checked out, it was research at the Memorial Sloan-Kettering Cancer Center in 1974 that at least in part confirmed the theory, even while MSKCC spokesmen continued to sing tenor roles in the Establishment chorus that forever damns Laetrile, Krebs, and the vitamin B_{17} theory of cancer induction and prevention.

In a report on "cyanonitriles" in 1974—and not released until December, 1976—MSKCC reported that Doctors Morton Schwartz, Jerome Nisselbaum, and Lloyd J. Old, Jr., had indeed found that selected animal and human cancers released cyanide from vitamin B_{17} compounds. A rabbit liver mixture liberated cyanide from both amygdalin and prunasin, four human liver samples released cyanide from prunasin, and five varieties of mouse tumors released cyanide from prunasin. Beta-glycosidases were the liberating enzymes.

A number of Laetrile researchers have speculated that prunasin—essentially amygdalin with only one sugar unit—may turn out to be more effective than amygdalin itself and that a synthetic prunasin, swiftly releasing its synergistic cyanide-benzaldehyde effect, might come closer than anything else to a "magic bullet" against cancer. By 1977, Israeli cancer researcher David Rubin, M.D., had announced dramatic anticancer results both with the use of large injectable levels of Laetrile (amygdalin) and with much smaller amounts of a Laetrile-like compound "biosynthesized" in the liver of goats from natural amygdalin. He told Michael L. Culbert that he had achieved the same anticancer effects of 70 grams of injectable Laetrile (amygdalin) with 2 or 3 grams of the biosynthesized material. These early results, and ongoing efforts in several quarters to find useful Laetrile-like derivatives, indicated that a potent synthetic Laetrile, perhaps along the lines of the product first developed by Ernst T. Krebs, Jr., will eventually emerge.

The only important aspect of the controversy is that vitamin B₁₇ *does* work, if by "work" we mean the variety of palliative effects ascribed to it, of which direct attack on cancer cells is only one. There has been a growing speculation that the raw natural foods containing vitamin B₁₇ may contain other elements that also work either on their own or in conjunction with B₁₇ itself as a prophylaxis against cancer. Apricot and peach kernels, for example, are abundant in potassium, which may be a "transporter" of cyanide into cells.

Krebs and other Beardians and modern researchers have now linked vitamin B₁₇, the *extrinsic* anticancer factor, with pancreatic enzymes and the body's immune system as the *intrinsic* anticancer factor, and in so doing have arrived at the following probable scenario for the nature and induction of cancer:

Let us say Joe Smith is a typical American male subsisting on a typical American diet. He is also a two-pack-a-day man. His continual smoking, through a variety of tissue abuse in the lungs, is setting up a constant irritation there. Joe drinks water containing carcinogens and breathes air polluted with lead and hydrocarbons. He eats an enormous amount of animal protein every day (eggs, other dairy products, red meat), and the protein-digesting enzymes of his pancreas are beginning to work overtime simply to keep up with their digestion duties.

Up to now, Joe has had cancer of the lungs *many* times— that is, estrogen has been activated during the involved process of tissue repair, primitive germ cells have been triggered into differentiation, and trophoblast may or may not have resulted. But each time the pancreatic enzymes, and perhaps other elements of the immune system, have been on hand to cut down this asexual new generation, this subclinical cancer, before it ever became noticeable. That is, the "first string" team was always there, doing its naturally selected job.

But now the tissues have been abused more and more by smoking. Joe is getting older and "slowing down," but his dietary habits are still those of a first-string quarterback. His pancreatic enzymes are spent in digestive activities. This time, a fresh irritation of the lungs has occurred, primitive germ cells have been activated, and trophoblast has been the result. *This* time, there are not sufficient pancreatic enzymes to do their job, or the pancreas itself is spent. And, most importantly, there is no "second string" team—no vitamin B_{17} compounds—because Joe's diet has virtually none of that life-saving material in it.

Without a first- or second-string team to do the job, the body reacts to the new entity as it does to an invader: it first surrounds the concentration of rapidly proliferating trophoblast with trophoblastlike tissue, as if in an effort to "trick" the trophoblast. It surrounds that tissue with natural tissue. The result is a lump or bump—or, in Joe's case, a "speck on the lung."

Ultimately, Joe's condition is diagnosed, and the worst is made known to him: *lung cancer.*

This scenario, repeated over and over again, may involve anybody and any tissue. The reaction of orthodox medicine to this now well-developed chain of events—frequently by the time an appearance is made by a cancer victim in a clinic the tumors have already vascularized and are developing their own blood supply—is to attack the resulting lump, bump, or speck as if *it* were the disease, and to attempt to cut it out, burn it, or poison it. Removal of the symptom, particularly at an early stage, and direct removal of the stimulus linked to the symptom (in Joe's case, giving up smoking) *may* have the effect of ending, at least for a while, the disease state that orthodoxy calls *cancer.* In more cases than not, however, the underlying, systemic, chronic cause of cancer (the weakness of the immune system or the utter lack of vitamin B_{17}) is by no means addressed and thus cancer will recur unless *another* degenerative Killer Disease, intercurrent with or developing faster than cancer—and also due to dietary deficiency or excess—occurs first and proves fatal.

We hasten to point out here that the Beardian theory on which Laetrile, or vitamin B_{17}, research was based is *not* vital to the question of whether vitamin B_{17} works or not, though it *is* important in assessing whether or not tests similar to the pregnancy test for women are indeed helpful in detecting subclinical cancer in men. (The human chorionic gonadotrophin hormone—HCG—is excreted in ever-increasing levels in both pregnancy and cancer. It should be noted that HCG production is the result of active cancer-cell metabolism but has no effects related to the production of cancer cells when injected into the body. It has been pointed out many times that cancer victims lose their appetite, and HCG from the urine of pregnant women has been used for many years as a method of treatment of obese patients to decrease appetite.)

The specific way in Laetrile works is not important when contrasted with the reality that it *does* work.

In light of the almost total failure of the orthodox War on Cancer, the billions of research dollars consumed in the search for the elusive "cancer-causing human virus" could better have been parlayed into investigating nutritional aspects of the disease and the now established records of B_{17}-based metabolic physicians who treat cancer. The combined Beardian–vitamin B_{17} theory of cancer induction comes nearer than any other to explaining the cause of cancer, and the B_{17}-based metabolic therapy program may at this time be a better approach than any other for dealing with a cancer crisis.

It comes closer than any other point of view in explaining how it is that whole groups of people, exposed to the same pollutants and contaminants as their neighbors, can avoid completely, or substantially, high levels of cancer. It explains why, on a farm, grazing animals are almost never seen with exhibitions of cancer, while domesticated cats and dogs, fed diets lacking in B_{17} foods which additionally have been treated with a number of chemicals suspected of cancer induction, may come down with cancer, as may the farmer and the farmer's family.

It successfully explains the raging pandemicity of cancer in the "civilized" Western world—one in which pollutants, contaminants, and poisons abound in the air, water, and food we consume, while at the same time we have virtually removed our natural defense against cancer from our food supply.

Indeed, failure to face this double reality means, morbidly enough, that there is little fear of overpopulation in the Western world—for, with time, "civilized" countries will be so decimated by cancer *alone* that overpopulation will not be a problem.

EMOTIONS

Information has slowly been developing that—quite aside from the overwhelming importance of nutrition and diet in cancer, and also quite aside from the ocean of carcinogens in which modern man struggles to survive—attitudes and emotions are linked to the onset of cancer, and doubtless may play a role in its prevention and treatment.

We will not involve ourselves here with "blue light" areas of the mystical, or the philosophical aspects of mind over matter, for this realm is far more speculative than corroborative. Yet data do exist to suggest links between how we think and the state of our health. The field for investigation into mental processes as inductors or collaborative inductors in disease is obviously wide open.

In 1976 Johns Hopkins University researchers released intriguing information on studies begun almost 30 years before: 1,337 medical students who entered Johns Hopkins between 1948 and 1964 were followed through their careers as students and doctors, with those surviving now ranging in age from 30 to 60.

In the Hopkins study, 41 of the doctors had died and 131 had fallen ill, including 16 listed as suicides. Illness patterns included 42 with cancer, 20 with high blood pressure, 14 with heart attacks, and 38 with mental illness.

The physicians who developed cancer had personality characteristics and family histories strikingly similar to those who became mentally ill or who committed suicide, the Hopkins researchers pointed out. These patterns included being low-keyed, quiet, emotional, self-contained, and lonely. As children they were not close to their parents. Indeed, noted researcher Dr. Caroline Bedell Thomas, the lack of closeness to family was "a striking and unexpected finding" in the study.

Nearly a third of the physicians who committed suicide, suffered cancer, or had mental illness indicated that their fathers were not steady, companionable, understanding, or warm, while less than 10 percent of all the students in the study had such fathers.

A task force of the American Psychological Association reported in 1975 that cancer often occurs in persons who repress unpleasant childhood experiences. Dr. David Kissen of the University of Glasgow, Scotland, found in a study of 150 lung cancer patients that such patients typically had difficulty expressing their emotions.

At the University of Rochester Medical Center in New York, psychiatrist Dr. William Greene found in a study of 100 men and women with two varieties of cancer—leukemia and lymphoma—that in all but a few cases the victims had suffered the loss of a loved one before developing this disease.

All of this is far too random and sketchy to be conclusive, but dim outlines of a "cancer personality" index do emerge. This is not to say that any such personality *will* develop cancer, but simply that the complex of emotions and attitudes involved *may* be involved with the body's reception to unchecked trophoblast. None of these traits can be determined as factors in babies or young children who are cancer-stricken.

It is of interest to a number of cancer specialists, however, that their patients may often express their mental attitudes in terms which may actually reflect the physical processes of cancer: "Something had been eating on me," "Something is gnawing at me," and "I'm keeping all this bottled up inside me" are such reflections.

At least one researcher has done well-documented work in using attitudes as part of the treatment of cancer. Dr. O. Carl Simonton, formerly chief of radiation therapy at Travis Air Force Base, California, reported in 1973 that in a two-year study of 152 cancer patients he had treated, he noted that the patients' improved or unimproved conditions correlated to their degree of participation in his special treatment program —which included meditation techniques—and to their positive or negative attitudes.

"The mind, the emotions, and the attitude of a patient play a role in both the development of a disease, cancer included, and the response that a patient has to any form of treatment," he said.

Dr. Simonton's interest in the attitudinal aspects of cancer had been spurred in 1969 at the University of Oregon Medical Center when he noted that certain patients "inexplicably" lived longer or were "unexpectedly" cured during radiation therapy—and that these were cancer sufferers who were beating enormous odds in advanced terminal cancer. In talking with these people Dr. Simonton consistently noted positive and stubborn attitudes such as "I can't die until such and such happens." These were people for whom cancer was utterly unexpected and absolutely unwanted—in contrast to those patients who, despite what they *said*, continued to flirt with death through what they *did:* those with lung cancer who continued to smoke, those with liver malignancy who went on drinking. Some of these patients said things like "Maybe I deserved this" or "It's probably punishment for what I did."

Dr. Simonton heard such patients describe their life situation at the time their cancers arose with such phrases as "I felt trapped" or "I hadn't much to live for." Very likely their subconscious minds had found a "way out" for them—cancer.

Andrew R. L. McNaughton, president-founder of the McNaughton Foundation, which for years was the only organization keeping interest in, and research on, Laetrile alive, assessed much the same situation when he wrote that "for many, cancer is a socially acceptable way of committing suicide."

We have observed this attitude in many cases. In interviews with hundreds of cancer patients, we have found that for many the diagnosis of cancer provokes a sigh of relief. Because cancer is so firmly riveted in the Western mind as synonymous with death, it represents, particularly for the religiously inclined, the certainty of death and the end to life's problems. For these individuals, who under Judaeo-Christian morality cannot consciously countenance the idea of suicide, cancer is the offer of relief through death.

Religious attitude *alone* has been seen time and again as a factor in control of cancer. Many patients, seeming to beat heavy odds against them, even temporarily, profess strong religious-faith patterns, and in the first series of interviews of 20 terminal cancer patients questioned for *Vitamin B17: Forbidden Weapon Against Cancer,* the faith-pattern level was very high in more than half the cases, even when death ultimately ensued, though always much beyond the general date that physicians had predicted.

Sensing that attitudes and emotions play a role in cancer induction, Dr. Simonton pioneered meditative techniques aimed at actual treatment of cancer. These involve the patient's "seeing" cancer in his mind's eye and visualizing the attack on it by lymphocytes. Patients were literally harangued into developing positive attitudes about themselves. Dr. Simonton reported impressive achievements for those who were attitudinally motivated and thus cooperated in the program, and much lower success rates for those who were less cooperative with the program.

However, far more work needs to be done before any specific statements on the harnessing of mental energy against cancer can be made definitively. At this time, the rule of thumb for cancer treatment would seem to be a total metabolic therapy program accompanied by the nurturing and encouragement of positive mental attitudes—for a holistic program cannot be "whole" unless the mind is involved.

BEATING CANCER THE NATURAL WAY

Despite the poison-laden, carcinogen-heavy milieu of Western civilization, the truth is that you do *not* need to fear cancer. Beating cancer the natural way necessarily falls into two parts: preventing it outright, and *treating* the condition, which is far and away the more complex of the two parts.

For all intents and purposes, cancer may be virtually eliminated in a single generation through the program we will outline. Prevention is, after all, the goal—but it is not the answer for the 675,000 new cases of cancer that will be diagnosed this year in the United States alone.

In terms of treatment, we stress, first and foremost, the extreme peril that a cancer patient will face should he attempt to treat himself. The reasons for this should be obvious: cancer is often intercurrent with other diseases or conditions, and only professional, competent diagnosis and follow-up can be relied upon to make such a determination. In addition, the metabolic treatment program suggested for cancer therapy will vary somewhat from patient to patient depending on individual needs and variances.

We have no doubt that a total metabolic program, emphasizing a radical change in eating habits, the administration of the "free-radical scavenger" vitamins A, C, and E, carefully coordinated dosages of vitamin B₁₇, and the administration of specific minerals, constitutes far and away the best path to follow in the treatment of this condition. But we also recognize that for about 95 percent of cancer patients it is almost certain that some orthodox course has already been followed —"heroic" surgery, chemotherapy and/or radiation.

There are times when surgery is an absolute necessity, as when a life-threatening tumor is encountered and there simply is not the time to wait for nutritional therapy to work, or when a tumor that has not metastasized can be excised without the sacrifice of large amounts of normal tissue and body defense mechanisms. The same may be true, from time to time, in the attempted radiation of life-threatening growths. But in the majority of cases, we contend that the greater the degree to which radiation and chemotherapy (the administration of toxic substances) are avoided, the greater are the chances that the cancer can be brought under control.

As we have pointed out, the real damage of chemotherapy and radiation is not so much to cancer cells as to normal tissue, inasmuch as even the great majority of a tumor mass is normal, or hostal, tissue, and the use of radiation or poison in the effort to get at the actual malignant cells is the equivalent of turning a blow torch on a wart. Worse, the body's immune system is so adversely affected by radiation and chemotherapy that in many cases it is not the cancer that kills the patient, but some minor infection that runs unchecked because the immune system cannot block it. In many instances, the orthodox treatment for cancer is worse than the disease itself.

We must add, for the millions who are under some kind of orthodox treatment, that there is absolutely nothing in the use of vitamin B₁₇ or vitamin therapy itself that is contraindicated or harmful when orthodox therapy is being used. Many patients have indeed been treated by mixtures of radiation, chemotherapy and the vitamin B₁₇ program. While this may not be advisable due to the tissue destruction of radiation and chemotherapy, there is absolutely no indication that natural therapy through vitamin B₁₇ cannot be successfully used with orthodox approaches. Indeed, we would add, if a patient is unable to come to terms with himself in seeking out the total metabolic program, vitamin B₁₇–based adjuvant therapy will at least have the effects of shoring up the immune system against the assault being made on it, and it may work both to counteract cancer-associated pain and to reduce or eliminate the dreadful side-effects of chemotherapy and radiation.

At this writing, medical staffs in the Tijuana clinics specializing in the Laetrile program were reporting a variety of successes by mixing orthodox with vitamin B_{17} treatment, particularly in being able to eliminate the nausea and associated general malaise which came from the use of chemotherapy, and being able to use small doses of chemotherapy after the administration of very large injections (9 to 12 grams intravenously per day) of Laetrile.

Again, we do not necessarily advise any such course of action. We mention this only to underscore the harmlessness of vitamin B_{17} and indeed the benign nature of *natural* therapy.

The treatment program for the metabolic control of cancer consists, as indicated, of the early and complete or almost complete elimination of animal proteins from the diet, even though the extent and length of this proscription are not universally agreed upon. Also banned are fatty foods and products made from refined white sugar and flour. Heavy emphasis is placed upon raw, fresh fruits and vegetables, their juices, and usually their seeds. The fresher the fruits and vegetables are and the more sprouted the natural grains and cereals, the better. While all red meat is banned, at least at the beginning of the program, some physicians allow limited amounts of fish and poultry. In order to supply the body with protein to build new normal cells through a balanced diet, the ingestion of liquid predigested protein (requiring no digestive work on the part of the pancreas) is frequently indicated.

There is a complete elimination of smoking and drinking and the avoidance of stimulants such as coffee and tea, though some herbal teas are permitted. Cola drinks, due to both their sugars and stimulants, are also expressly forbidden.

To the extent that it is possible, we suggest that cancer patients avoid all artificially colored and flavored foods and as much processed food as possible. We know this is a tall order, particularly in an urban setting, but natural, organically grown fruits and vegetables are superior to the nutrition-stripped, colored, sweetened, emulsified, or otherwise tampered-with foods that have gone through processing.

In terms of *hygiene,* it is recommended that cancer patients not be in close or unventilated rooms with smokers, that they increase their oxygen intake with open-air exercises every day and as far away as possible from known sources of pollution, that they take daily warm baths, evacuate their bowels at least once a day, sleep a good eight or nine hours daily, and avoid permanent-wave lotions, toxic hair sprays, synthetic cosmetics, antiperspirants, and lipsticks made out of coal-tar dyes. Some metabolic therapists insist on daily enemas, including coffee enemas (excellent detoxifiers of the liver) in order to cleanse the system, while others believe that the radical change in diet and the use of specific vitamins will accomplish the needed detoxification.

In line with both the trophoblastic theory and the clinical evidence from using them on their own merits as cancer-killers, pancreatic enzymes and allied protein-digesting (proteolytic) enzymes are usually also administered in the metabolic treatment of cancer. The thinking here is that the administration of these substances will assist in the digestion of protein—something the overworked pancreas normally does along with maintaining an intrinsic surveillance against trophoblast, or cancer—and will also attack the trophoblast. The natural pancreatic enzymes and their manufactured homologues help "de-shield" the trophoblasts, or cancer cells, leaving them open to attack by white blood cells, and may do some of the attacking themselves.

Used in this regard are the Wobe-Mugos enzymes, technically illegal in the U.S. and pioneered in West Germany, and Viokase and Pancreatin, a product of E. Lilly and Company. Bromelain, a proteolytic enzyme produced from pineapples, is also useful and frequently employed in the total therapy.

Vitamins A, C, and E are also routinely prescribed in the total therapy. Vitamin A, already shown to have inhibited carcinogen and virus-connected tumors in laboratory animals, has become increasingly linked with cancer prevention and treatment, particularly in West German experiments. Since it is largely found in its natural state in animal tissue in nature, and because most animal products are banned from the cancer treatment program, vitamin A is useful simply as a supplement to make up for a probable deficiency in the diet, one also brought about because plant-source vitamin A must

169

be produced from carotene, the amount of which in many foods is low and variable. Weight loss, inappetence (loss of appetite) and increased susceptibility to infections have been laid to vitamin A deficiency as well. Despite the expressed concerns of American medical orthodoxy over alleged toxicity from vitamin A, many physicians use up to 200,000 units (or more under close supervision) per day in cancer patients with good results, and there are only a few recorded cases in which vitamin A "overdoses" caused distress to patients. Zinc and vitamin E have been found helpful in aiding the body's absorption and utilization of vitamin A.

Vitamin C, a potent antioxidant, has been found useful in the fight against cancer in megadoses, and has resulted in some cases in the outright control of cancer, as seen in the work of Stone, Pauling, and Cameron. It is also implicit in the strengthening of collagen, the "cement" between epithelial cells. Along with vitamin E and vitamin B_{15}, vitamin C is an excellent chelating agent—that is, these vitamins help to remove unwanted substances deposited inside cells and on the arterial walls, thus aiding in the increase of circulation and providing more oxygen and other nutrients to individual cells. Vitamin C is given therapeutically at anywhere from 5,000 mg per day and up—with some cases on record of dose levels as high as 50 grams. Megadoses given by mouth may cause diarrhea or irritate an existing ulcer in the stomach.

Vitamin E, an excellent antioxidant as well as a mild chelating agent, is also useful together with selenium in maintaining cellular wall integrity and in helping the body produce more antibodies to head off various invaders. Therefore, vitamin E and selenium are excellent protection against carcinogens. As with vitamin C, no overdose has been known to occur. Vitamin E complements the action of vitamin B_{15} and also helps the absorption of vitamin A. It is suggested that only the *d-alpha* variety as acetate or succinate be used. Vitamin E is being confirmed as such an excellent metabolic agent for a wide variety of conditions that its use is widely indicated across the board, except in some cases of excessively high blood pressure or when the blood pressure elevates after ingestion of vitamin E. One to six 400 IU capsules per day are suggested.

Multiple vitamins are also used. Any of several commercial preparations available, particularly those including the full B complex (that is, the B chain normally recognized up to, but not including, B_{15} and B_{17}), may be used in the total program, since such preparations may provide missing nutrients whose lack or deficiencies have not otherwise been noted.

Vitamin B_{15}, or pangamic acid, which many metabolic therapists believe may constitute a discovery of more far-reaching significance than vitamin B_{17}, since its usefulness and effects are of an apparently very wide span, greatly aids the provision of oxygen to the cancer cell, a cell whose "reverse chemistry" is marked by aversion to oxygen and metabolism through fermentation. At the same time, B_{15} increases the oxygen supply to normal cells. All clinical conditions marked by impairment in metabolism, muscle contraction and cellular permeability are considered targets for B_{15} use. It is regarded as a considerable methylating agent that helps to spark the synthesis of phosphocreatine, an element common to membrane permeability, muscle contraction, and nerve conduction.

It is an interesting side note that the Soviet Union has reported on and advanced vitamin B_{15} therapy and its use in athletes. The Russians actually "lifted" the idea from Ernst T. Krebs, Jr. The American Medical Association seems to have "discovered" vitamin B_{15} on the basis of the research work done by the Russians, while the same American medical elite continues to denounce Krebs as a quack.

American researchers have noted that B_{15} is of great benefit to those who live in areas high in air pollution and that it has been found useful in treating cirrhosis of the liver and hepatitis. Its detoxifying ability makes it of probable benefit in the treatment for poisoning from alcohol, drugs, and chemicals. Some Soviet researchers have claimed that diabetes can be cured with B_{15}, and it has been found useful in treating hypertension, asthma, neuritis, dermatitis, early stages of cataracts and glaucoma, arthritis, male infertility, sciatica, and early stages of gangrene.

A water-soluble substance, B_{15} is naturally found in seeds, nuts, brewer's yeast, and animal organs. There is no known overdose or toxicity from pangamic acid, and starting therapy is usually 150 mg per day, or three 50 mg capsules. Dosage levels must be suited to individual needs, and levels may exceed 500 mg per day.

Minerals are routinely provided in cancer cases after ade-

171

quate diagnosis, either for mineral imbalance or the existence of mineral toxicities, usually traced through hair analysis. Quantitative analysis of hair becomes valuable since the body excretes minerals through the fingernails and hair. (The process is explained in chapter three.)

Of frequent use are calcium, magnesium, and zinc as orotates. The body's absorption of minerals is in direct proportion to the amount of minerals present in the intestinal tract as well as the absorbability (absorption factor) of the minerals themselves. The positively charged ions tend to be "bound" by the cells of the intestinal tract. Therefore, one of the primary ways of increasing the absorption of minerals from the intestinal tract is to "bind" the mineral with a protein molecule and thus permeability and absorbability of the mineral are increased since the ionic charge of the mineral is no longer present and therefore the mineral is not bound on the cells of the lining of the intestinal tract. The minerals with a protein molecule become absorbed as if they were proteins and can be better utilized and better transferred across the cellular membranes of the organs of the body.

One of the most effective protein molecules for binding calcium, magnesium, and zinc is that of orotatic acid, a product of milk whey. The minerals are "bonded" chemically with the molecule of orotatic acid and thus produce calcium, magnesium, and zinc orotates. There are various other amino acids (protein molecules) that are of value in binding different mineral molecules, thus increasing their absorbability from the intestinal tract and also assisting their transfer across cellular membranes within the body.

Calcium orotate is useful in the protection of vital structures from immune system attack, in recalcification of bone metastases, and for treatment of decalcification caused by cortisone and X-ray treatment. Magnesium orotate is useful in the dilation of blood vessels and in regenerating damaged liver tissue. The minerals help to relieve pain and reduce anxiety.

It should be noted that magnesium is used in more than 75 percent of the enzyme reactions in the body. There are over 5,300 known enzyme systems, a good number of which produce many different kinds of enzyme molecules that have specific reactions within cells in order to maintain a normal metabolic condition.

Zinc is used in the healing of damaged cells and in the repair of damaged or injured tissue. It is used in the body to cause a rapid proliferation of new normal tissue. Zinc is also of primary importance in the production of insulin, the hormone produced by the pancreas, which, as we have seen, is essential to the control of blood sugar levels within the body.

Vitamin B_{17} (amygdalin, Laetrile) is considered the crown jewel in the cancer-treatment diadem because it is, aside from collateral functions, apparently cancer-specific. Injections of Laetrile in "terminal" cases, gradually replaced by Laetrile tablets, form the center of the total metabolic treatment approach, and it is current thinking that since cancer reflects a specific deficiency in vitamin B_{17}, the patient should stay on maintenance levels of the substance for the remainder of his life.

The normal period for the crash treatment of a "terminal cancer crisis" is about three to four weeks, though it may be longer. During this time, the radically altered diet, accompanied by the use of proteolytic enzymes, other vitamins, and minerals, is commenced along with injections of Laetrile, usually intravenously. It is safe to say that Laetrile exerts a broad variety of effects on the patients aside from the unleashing of cancer-fighting agents through the breaking down of amygdalin into cyanide and benzaldehyde. Some of these effects are often dramatic, and almost immediate, and involve the decrease or elimination of the pain associated with cancer (but not with anything else), a stimulus to appetite, weight gain, restoration of natural color, and an improved disposition.

For years, beginning dosages of 3 grams intravenously daily, gradually changing to intravenous injections every other day and to tablets on alternate days, and then to a maintenance level of tablets only, was the standard Laetrile therapy, generally accompanied by a vigorous dietary program and the use of other vitamins and proteolytic enzymes. However, 1975 and 1976 marked the general use of 9 grams intravenously per day, and by 1977 as much as 12 grams intravenously daily was being used in the early treatment stage. Some physicians have used as high as 70 grams intravenously daily in beginning treatment without toxic side-effects.

Laetrile is, again, so essentially nontoxic that its upper levels of potential use are not known. Some of the elements that Laetrile-using physicians watch for in the course of treatment are the possible lowering of blood pressure due to the metabolites of free cyanide, which help form thiocyanate which in turn may lower blood pressure, and body reactions to the toxic by-products of the destruction of cancerous, or trophoblastic, cells. In some cases, the destruction of the malignancy is so rapid that the body cannot detoxify fast enough, and fever, dizziness, edema, vertigo, and general malaise may temporarily result. The response here is to lower the dosage temporarily, but any such effects are positive in that they indicate that the treatment is working.

Following three to four weeks of injection-based Laetrile therapy, patients then begin alternating tablets with shots and gradually may be moved onto a tablet-only B_{17} regimen, on which they are urged to remain for the rest of their lives along with foods that are high in B_{17}.

It is vital to reemphasize that the measurement of palpable lumps and bumps—the "index of tumefaction"—is *not* a part of the natural, metabolic program in cancer treatment. Indeed, as was noted earlier, in many cases of metabolic treatment, one early reaction may very well be that there are *more* tumors than before. But again, this is a positive sign that the body's immune system is being stimulated to help ward off cancer. Remember, the majority of the mass in most tumors is natural tissue, and the formation of tumors represents the body's response to cancer, or trophoblast, so a temporary sudden increase in tumors is not generally a cause for alarm under the vitamin B_{17} program.

The B_{17}-based management of cancer is, after all, a total metabolic treatment program for the whole body, and is *not* an attack on tumors alone. The substances administered are providing needed nutrition to the body so that cell metabolism can return to normal, and so that the immune system can be shored up, making it possible for the body to fight the condition. This is a revolutionary departure from the use of toxic chemicals and radiation to poison, burn, or blast out tumors, and not only does *not* harm the natural tissue, but actually strengthens the body and provides a specific assault on cancer.

The B_{17} management program does not guarantee a cure for cancer, nor do metabolic therapists who use this program offer any such cure. At the very best, the B_{17} program offers a control for cancer, in the same way that the relevant vitamins offer controls (but not cures) for pellagra, pernicious anemia, beriberi, rickets, and scurvy.

The great majority of patients in the United States who turn to the metabolic management of cancer, unfortunately, are usually "terminal." This may mean that their cancers are regarded as irreversible, that their cancers have done so much damage that the individual is not expected to survive, *or* that they are dying because of the horrendous effects of standard, orthodox treatment.

For the majority of these people who *are* seeking, desperately, a magical guaranteed cure, the metabolic program can offer little more than a wide range of palliation, and, even then, only in a majority of—but by no means in all—cases. Even a widespread attack on cancer cells themselves, to the point where cancer is itself stopped in its tracks, cannot restore the lost or damaged tissue, which loss and/or damage may still prove fatal to the patient. And, certainly, the wholesale destruction of natural tissue by orthodox treatment cannot be reversed by a last-ditch turning to the total metabolic program.

A general pattern is that the sooner one turns to the total metabolic program for cancer, the more likely his success in beating the disease and the more certain his recovery, but that recovery is not due simply to finding a physician who will administer Laetrile injections, for the intravenous administration of vitamin B_{17} is only part of the program, and when used by itself it is almost never successful.

In the 1970s, Laetrile researchers were pointing with enthusiasm to a handful of cases which indicated some striking cancer control simply through the use of natural vitamin B_{17} sources themselves, primarily apricot and peach kernels, consumed in amounts of anywhere from 50 to over 100 per day. In three cases made known to Dr. Ernst T. Krebs, Jr., the use of the kernels was virtually the only anticancer therapy being used. The possibility loomed that, with time and research, reliance on the natural sources alone, in adequate amounts, might supplant the use of injectable and tablet material (which is, again, nothing more than refined amygdalin), at least in many cases of cancer. Part of the reason for the striking effects from use of the raw material itself is doubtless due to the fact that the kernels and seeds themselves are loaded with a host of substances, of which vitamin B_{17} (which comprises up to 3 percent of an apricot or peach kernel) is only one, and which may work better in unison with other substances, and/or be of only auxiliary importance to some other substance or chemical interchange not yet suspected by clinicians.

Along with the total metabolic treatment program, most physicians stress the role of mental attitude as essential— sometimes *equally* essential—in therapy. Encouraging and shoring up a positive mental attitude used to be part and parcel of the "bedside manner" for which the home-visiting general practitioners of days long gone were so prized. Indeed, this gentle psychological manipulation, so inherent a part of the *art*—rather than the mechanical craft—of medicine, is one of the most outstanding of the missing features of modern crisis, fragmented, specialized, or assembly-line medicine.

The person who does not wish to live, and for whom cancer is a convenient way out, or who mistakenly believes that cancer always means death, and who is not stimulated to undertake the discipline for the implicit change in lifestyle called for by total metabolic therapy, manifestly does less well than does the cheerful patient with a bright outlook and combative spirit, and it is up to the physician, at least in part, to stimulate, encourage, and nurture such an attitude.

"How do I know if I have cancer?" This is a naturally recurring question in a civilization justifiably in a panic over the growing incidence of the disease.

It is quite true that any of cancer's danger signs, as so outlined by the American Cancer Society (change in bowel or bladder habits, a sore that does not heal, unusual bleeding or discharge, thickening or lump in the breast or elsewhere, indigestion or difficulty in swallowing, obvious change in a wart or mole, nagging cough or hoarseness), are useful in bringing the possibility of cancer to the attention of a doctor. But unfortunately, by the time cancer is diagnosed under orthodoxy, chances are excellent that it has already spread from one tissue to another—and therefore that the victim is already well on the way to being considered terminal.

Cancer diagnostic tools have been developed that are as "outside the pale" as is Laetrile itself, but one of them in particular is beginning to achieve some positive recognition from Establishment medicine. While certainly imperfect, it constitutes, at this time, the best *early detection* test for the reaction of the body to malignancy, and not so coincidentally, it is in complete alignment with the trophoblastic theory of cancer.

While routinely used by Laetrile-dispensing physicians in several countries, until recently this particular test was damned as out-and-out quackery, primarily because it has nothing to do with "lumps and bumps." But it is frequently able to detect cancer at the preclinical level.

The test in question is the detection of human chorionic gonadtrophin (HCG), a hormone known to be secreted by pregnant women, and whose use was first advanced in a specific way by such scientists as Dr. Howard Beard of Texas (no relation to embryologist John Beard) as the Beard Anthrone Test (BAT), and which was refined to a claimed higher degree of accuracy by oncologist and medical researcher Manuel D. Navarro, M.D., at the University of Santo Tomás, Manila, Philippines, who is now recognized as the major world expert on the HCG test. Dr. Navarro has been using HCG detection in cancer since 1963, and has written extensively on the subject.

That HCG might be detected equally in the urine of pregnant mothers as well as of cancer-stricken men—men who even, at the time, had no other outward sign of the disease—flows quite naturally from the hypothesis that cancer *is* trophoblast at the wrong time and/or place; that is, the body reacts to the asexual extrauterine preembryo (cancer) the way it reacts to the developing embryo. HCG, which is broken up by the pancreatic enzyme chymotrypsin (a specific enzyme implicit in the destruction of trophoblast), is known to rise in the urine of the pregnant woman until the fifty-sixth day of pregnancy (the commencing function of the fetal pancreas) when it begins to decline, but it rises steadily in the urine of cancer patients until death.

By 1971, Navarro and his associates had detected HCG in the urine of 1,563 cases of proven cancers located from head to toe and belonging to 34 different histological (tissue) types, including leukemia. Largely laughed at by orthodoxy for arguing repeatedly in medical journals that the HCG "immunoassay" used for detecting pregnancies could also detect cancer, Navarro and the HCG test backers received some unexpected support from within orthodoxy in the United States.

177

First, in 1969 J. E. Dailey and P. M. Marcuse reported the probable aid from HCG detection in diagnosing lung cancer and suggested that the use of "more sensitive techniques . . . for chorionic gonadotrophin might lead to the diagnosis of more patients with bronchogenic carcinoma while they are still amenable to treatment."

Then, in 1973 a National Institute of Health team reported the presence of HCG in a substantial number of patients with a variety of tumors.

In 1976, Dr. Judith L. Vaitukaitis, of the Boston University School of Medicine, reported that HCG appeared to be an effective "marker" for a wide variety of tumors, including adenocarcinomas of the stomach, ovary, and pancreas, as well as hepatomas.

The *Medical Tribune Report,* as if totally unaware of the years of experience already reported by Navarro and his colleagues, recorded: "She [Dr. Vaitukaitis] said that radioactively labeled HCG can be detected in the blood . . . of patients with many types of tumor but not in normal persons, except for pregnant women. Since the radioimmunoassay was developed about three years ago, Dr. Vaitukaitis has found that the level of HCG correlates well with the course of breast cancer and is an exceptionally sensitive marker for gestational trophoblastic disease."

The interpretation here might be that HCG levels are detectable in the urine or blood of patients whose cancers exhibit trophoblastic involvement—an involvement in some cancer not denied by orthodoxy. But what if *all* cancer *is* trophoblastic, as the Beardians postulate? Then HCG detection itself may be construed as a detection for cancer per se.

Exciting possibilities in a one-minute blood test developed in England loomed on the diagnostic front in 1976. A test in which white blood cells are isolated from the blood and mixed with protein tissue taken from known cancer patients and examined with special instruments using polarized light showed a success rate of 97 percent among 700 human volunteers in diagnosing early-stage cancer and pinpointing its location. The diagnostic test developed by Boris and Lea Cercek at Patterson Research Institute in Manchester, and confirmed by laboratories in Japan, Germany, and Wales, may be given repeatedly and does not entail the dangers inherent in X-ray examinations or biopsies—diagnostic tools of choice that in some cases have actually helped spread the disease.

Let us point out here and strongly emphasize that nobody should rely simply on the early diagnosis of cancer. The reliance should be on *prevention*. One should spend far less energy in detecting cancer than he spends on *preventing* it. But between the two worlds—the speculative world of total prevention of cancer through natural means on the one hand, and the orthodox world of diagnosing lumps and bumps and then treating these symptoms on the other—the HCG detection test seems, at this time, the best diagnostic tool available, particularly since it gives indication of trophoblastic activity well in advance of any of "cancer's seven warning signals."

It is our assertion that vitamin B_{17}–based total metabolic therapy is the best *treatment* for cancer—that a cancer victim's odds for beating this major killer are much better under metabolic and nutritional management than under the auspices of standard therapy. But even so, *treatment* is a long way from the guarantee of victory over cancer, or the elimination, for all practical purposes, of this scourge of Western civilization.

Prevention is the key, and it is in the area of prevention wherein the B_{17}-centered approach achieves its highest success quotients. With adequate levels of vitamin B_{17} restored to the diet, together with the return of more biologically rational eating habits, cancer could be virtually eliminated in a single generation.

We have pointed to the "prudent diet" already advanced for prevention of heart disease—less animal protein, less fat, less starch, and less processed carbohydrates—and to the "food-for-life" diet in chapter five as useful to cancer prevention. With less reliance on processed foods, more ingestion of fruits and vegetables *and their seeds,* more natural grains and cereals, and with more foods in their raw or sprouting stages, we have the background for a healthy diet aimed at warding off degenerative disease and slowing down the aging process.

We would now add the utterly essential restoration of vitamin B_{17} to one's daily diet as the sine qua non of a virtually guaranteed life without cancer. However, we have to attach some explanations here.

A "recommended daily allowance" for vitamin B_{17} has not been set and is not even known, not only because standard nutrition has not yet generally recognized the nitrilosides, or cyanophoric glycosides, as a vitamin, but also because precise research and information are lacking. Both these lacks could be more than overcome if a modest amount of the tax and private money funneled into either the War on Cancer or the American Cancer Society was diverted into this obviously crucial area. But as of this writing no such efforts have been made.

Furthermore, we cannot make the blanket statement that a certain amount of vitamin B_{17} in the diet will absolutely protect against cancer if the individual continues to abuse his tissues (by chain-smoking and/or habitual drinking, for example), though the indications are indeed strong that sufficient vitamin B_{17}, for most people, might more than offset some bad habits. Prudence dictates that *every* effort be made in terms of more rational eating habits and less abusive lifestyles to accompany the return of vitamin B_{17} in the diet as nature's best protection against the cancer slaughter.

We also differentiate between the cancer-*prevention* diet and the cancer-*treatment* diet. The prevention diet is simply the food-for-life diet (see chapter five) *plus* the willful addition of vitamin B_{17}. This means less red meat, more fruits and vegetables (preferably as raw and fresh as possible, and preferably organically grown), more natural whole grains and cereals, and the consumption of at least some of the seeds in most fruits that are consumed. Greater avoidance of processed white sugar and processed white flour and their products is a necessary part of this general diet, along with a reduction in stimulants, smoking, and drinking. We have said reduction, not elimination, although a strict avoidance of such noxious habits will afford an ever greater degree of security.

Making use of a high-quality juicer can be of great help in preparing liquid preparations of fruits and vegetables, though one should be careful not to use a centrifugal juicer since it may destroy some naturally occurring enzymes.

Despite the fact that modern food processing and Western dietary habits have virtually eliminated vitamin B_{17} from our ingestion patterns, the vitamin remains ubiquitous in nature and may be easily obtained.

It naturally occurs in the seeds of every fruit grown in North America with the exception of the citrus fruits, and in these seeds, as well as the bitter almond (not to be confused with the sweet almond, which does not contain B$_{17}$), we find the highest known concentrations of the substance. A bite into an apple seed will produce a mild, slightly bitterish taste, which is the hallmark of natural vitamin B$_{17}$. It is the bitterness of the natural food source, paralleled by the West's gradual addiction to sugar and palate dependence on sweet-tasting foods largely devoid of nutrients, that accounts for sociological rejection of much of vitamin B$_{17}$ from the diet.

The known sources of vitamin B$_{17}$, and there are probably many others, include:

Kernels or seeds of fruit: the highest concentrations of vitamin B$_{17}$, aside from bitter almonds—apricot, peach, pear, plum, prune, apple, cherry and nectarine seeds.

Beans: broad (*Vicia faba*), burma, chickpeas, lima, Rangoon, scarlet runner, lentil (sprouted), mung (sprouted).

Nuts: bitter almond, macadamia, cashew.

Berries: almost all wild berries—blackberry, chokeberry, Christmasberry, cranberry, elderberry, raspberry, strawberry.

Seeds: chia, flax, sesame.

Grasses: acacia, aquatic, Johnson, milkweed, Sudan, tunus, velvet, wheat grass, white clover, alfalfa (sprouted).

Grains: millet, barley, oat and buckwheat groats, brown unpolished rice, chia, flax, rye, vetch, wheat berries.

Miscellaneous: bamboo shoots, fuchsia plant, sorghum, wild hydrangea, yew tree (needles, fresh leaves), manioc (cassava).

The possible uses of any or all of the above in a variety of ways should be obvious, for many of these items still exist in Western eating habits and are easily placed in family menus —everything from buckwheat pancakes to elderberry brandy, from salads enriched with garbanzos (chickpeas) to Chinese dinners with bamboo shoots and soups with lentils. Even so, we are dealing with minimal amounts of vitamin B$_{17}$, and no one is suggesting the consumption of several pounds of lima beans at a sitting.

The amount of vitamin B$_{17}$ in any of the sources will depend on many factors, but the easiest and surest way to guarantee a high concentration of the material is the ingestion of fruit seeds, particularly apricot and peach kernels, and also, for the sake of convenience, apple seeds.

To the Western palate, so habituated to sweet-tasting pulpy

foods, the bitterness of the apricot and peach kernel, or of the other seeds, is the first barrier to the most certain natural approach to the restoration of vitamin B_{17} at important levels. Yet, within a short period of time, many consumers develop a fondness for these seeds, and such diverse peoples as the Hunzakuts of Asia and several North American Indian tribes have long prized such nitrilosidic seeds and consumed them as snacks or prepared tea from them.

For those for whom bitterness is a continuing problem, we point out that the seeds are easily consumed by grinding them up as a fine powder, using them in salads, as part of a salad dressing, or with morning oatmeal.

Laetrile researchers have developed at least two rules of thumb in approaching an answer to the most oft-asked question: How many apricot or peach kernels should I eat to prevent cancer? Neither rule of thumb is a confirmed scientific fact, but the following of either is in accord with biological wisdom, and, as far as the authors can determine, neither has ever been disproved.

(1) Eat as many seeds of the fruits involved as you would if you were eating the whole fruits themselves. That is, a biologically rational amount of vitamin B_{17} is obtained from apple seeds eaten from the same number of apples that you might reasonably consume on any given day—if three apples, then the seeds of three apples, but not the equivalent of fifty apples' worth of seeds. That is logic and simplicity itself, for nature *is* logical and simple.

(2) It is theorized that more than sufficient vitamin B_{17} for cancer prevention is obtainable in most cases by the consumption of one apricot or peach kernel per 10 pounds of body weight. For a 170-pound man, that would mean 17 kernels, divided into three portions per day. Some speculators argue that this amount on alternate days is sufficient; others feel that double the amount would be better.

Following either rule of thumb, we assert, is the best single action the reader can take to afford himself of a natural vitamin B_{17} defense against the onset of cancer.

The Food and Drug Administration and state boards of medical health licensure began alerting citizens as early as 1974 to alleged dangers lurking in the consumption of apricot kernels due to the fact that active vitamin B_{17} contains a unit of cyanide. Indeed, the cyanide scare was heightened in 1976 to induce state agents to pressure health food store operators from storing packaged, prepitted apricot kernels, and earlier, to ban the Laetrile-containing food products Aprikern and Bee Seventeen. In the matter of the latter, millions of packets and capsules were sold—with no reported side-effects, let alone fatalities—before the FDA ban. In the matter of the former, law enforcement has relied on some extremely sketchy and at times "anecdotal" evidence, usually from foreign sources, to claim toxicity from the consumption of apricot kernels and also from other cyanophoric glycoside-containing plants such as cassava. The toxicity studies from the United States, which consist of less than a half-dozen cases, none of them fatal, involve individuals consuming unusually large amounts of kernels and usually ingesting them after doing irrational things—such as, in one case, grinding up hundreds in a blender, and leaving them standing in water in an open container on a windowsill all night.

It is true that an individual may consume too much or too many of anything, including water, and this is true for apricot (or peach, plum, pear or apple) kernels as well. We can speculate that many hundreds of the kernels forced into the empty stomach of an adult with lots of water added might produce some cyanide toxicity. The fact is, of course, that any unreasonable action, such as the introduction of a thimbleful of water into a lung, or a bubble of air into a vein, will produce a fatal side-effect. And it *may* be true that some populations with very high concentrations of cyanophoric glycoside foods, to the exclusion of many other foods, *may* have suffered some side-effects. But there simply is no evidence to suggest that reasonable amounts of apricot kernels consumed under reasonable conditions provide anything other than excellent nutrition for the body.

The scare tactics arrayed against vitamin B_{17}–containing foods are based on the word *cyanide*. It is true that free cyanide is a deadly poison. But the cyanide in B_{17} compounds is not free. It is a cyanide radical naturally bound with other elements in a sugar compound. The natural seeds do contain the enzymes that may "unlock" the natural cyanide, so that whatever danger may lurk in a premature "unlocking" is true for the natural source of Laetrile, not the refined product (concentrated amygdalin) itself, which has been used in doses as high as 100 grams daily topically and up to 70 grams daily intravenously without any known toxic side-effects.

Apricot and peach kernels, after all, are God's natural tablets. Not only are they heavily laden with amygdalin, in amounts ranging up to 3 percent each, but they are also very abundant in calcium, magnesium, sodium, and potassium, and carry some amount of iron, copper, manganese, and zinc. They are, then, simply *good food*.

That government forces would move to confiscate apricot kernels on the basis of alleged toxicity, while allowing over-the-counter sales of aspirin, fatal to well over 100 babies per year, is only evidence of the continuing efforts by vested interests to "get at" Laetrile, the natural health foods, and the theory and practice of preventive medicine. Some of the repression may be due to the box that orthodoxy had put itself into by the mid-1970s; while admitting that the product Laetrile itself is nontoxic, it struck out at the natural raw material for it (in North America), even though it takes many hundreds of apricot kernels' worth of amygdalin to fill a normal vial of amygdalin.

It is often asked if cooking will destroy vitamin B_{17} in seeds and vegetables or somehow liberate the safely bound cyanide molecule. The answer is no. Vegetables cooked at the same temperature as a Chinese dinner will not lose their healthy B_{17} content, even though the "unlocking enzyme," beta-glucosidase, may be burned off, causing a more complicated release of the vitamin B_{17} elements. There is no good substitute for the natural ingestion of B_{17} in its natural state—the eating and chewing of the raw material, with which man evolved for millions of years, in distinction to the 10,000 or so years he may have engaged in cooking.

Fears of cyanide aside (and, under appropriate conditions, cyanide can be "liberated" from roast beef, gelatin, and lettuce, yet no campaign against these foods has been attempted), vitamin B_{17} is a natural, normal part of the scheme of things. Man evolved in an ambience in which vitamin B_{17} played a natural role, an environment in which at least 1,400 natural sources of the material were available to him. This same environment still exists for wild range animals—in which no malignancies are ever found—and even for the domesticated grazing animals whose natural foods consist of heavily nitrilosidic grasses, a natural vegetation that protects them against cancer.

FIVE

"You Are What You Eat"

FOOD FOR LIFE

It is the central thesis of this book that to be healthy and to prevent degenerative diseases it is necessary that the right amount of the right nutrients be at the right place at the right time and in the right proportion to other nutrients. Unfortunately, this is not always possible for the average American in spite of the claims of medical and nutritional orthodoxy that we are the best fed nation in the world.

The fallacy of this position is explained by Dr. Roger Williams in *Nutrition Against Disease:* "The orthodox position advanced in medical education today appears to be this: 'The blood routinely carries full nourishment to all the cells and tissues.' This is preposterous biologically; it overlooks the crucial, undeniable fact that whether the blood carries adequate nutrition or not *depends upon what we eat.*"

Part of this way of thinking was beginning to make itself heard as 1977 opened. The Senate Select Committee on Nutrition and Human Needs report warned that Americans must make drastic changes in their eating habits if they want to live longer.

The panel's report, "Dietary Goals for the United States," argued for reduction in the consumption of things Americans love to eat and drink—soft drinks, candy, baked goods, potato chips, pretzels, and red meat.

Senator George McGovern, the committee's chairman, told a news conference that "too much fat, too much sugar or salt can be and are linked directly to heart disease, cancer, obesity and stroke, among other killer diseases."

The report, which called for increasing the consumption of fruits, vegetables, and whole grain products, while reducing sugar by 40 percent, salt by 50 to 85 percent, and fat by 10 percent, was doubly significant in that it was the first by any government body to offer specific recommendations for changing dietary habits.

Obviously, any diet not prepared for a specific individual cannot take into account specific individual needs. However, assuming that you are not being treated dietetically for some problem, there are some suggestions we can make that will improve your nutritional intake.

(1) Avoid processed foods in which there are food dyes, additives, preservatives, sugar, or white flour. Included here are the so-called convenience foods such as processed cereal, all substitute breakfast drinks like Tang and Instant Breakfast, TV dinners, all bread except 100 percent stone-ground whole grain varieties, and anything else that has sugar, white flour, or any kind of preservatives and/or additives. As is correctly pointed out in *Psychodietetics,* "Supermarket shelves are packed full of incredible edibles, more toys than real foods. *Quick, ee-zee* or *redi,* they have a nutritional content as atrocious as their spelling."

(2) Eat only lean meats and remove any strips of fat before cooking. Try to avoid eating beef more than two or three times a week and have more of other lean meats as well as organ meats (heart, liver, brains, sweetbreads, et cetera) and seafood and poultry.

The sweeteners and nitrates and nitrites may be removed from processed meats such as ham, bacon, and luncheon meats by immersing the product in boiling water. To completely remove them, the meat should be immersed in two separate pots of boiling water for one minute each.

(3) Eggs may be eaten in moderate amounts and need not be limited to three a week as some have mistakenly advocated because of the cholesterol content. Most of the cholesterol in the bloodstream is manufactured by the body, and even if no cholesterol is eaten, arteriosclerosis may still result. Cholesterol levels are kept in check not by the amount of cholesterol one eats but by such things as lecithin, vitamin B₃ and vitamin C. Eggs contain lecithin as well as other vital nutrients; therefore, eliminating eggs from one's diet is not

only unnecessary, but it is also unwise from a nutritional point of view.

(4) Natural hard cheese and cottage cheese in its natural state are good sources of protein that can be eaten as snacks as well as with meals.

(5) Salt-free, unroasted nuts, sunflower seeds, and apricot and peach kernels are also good sources of protein and other nutrients, and can be eaten as snacks.

(6) Vegetables, especially green leaf and green stalk vegetables, are an important part of any eating program. They should be eaten as fresh as possible and either raw or cooked only until they are crisp, as in the Japanese manner. Vegetable juices may be made by placing vegetables in a blender.

(7) Fresh fruit and fruit juices should be consumed daily without any sweeteners. If you are addicted to sweet tastes, use only artificial sweeteners.

Fruit and vegetable juices are sources of immediate energy upon arising in the morning. If additional protein is desired, a protein powder of not less than 90 percent protein and *no* carbohydrates along with one teaspoon of brewer's yeast flakes may be added to the juice and mixed in a blender. A raw egg may also be added if desired.

(8) Whole grain cereals and 100 percent stone-ground whole grain breads, preferably of the mixed-grain variety, may be eaten so long as there are no additives or sugar in them.

(9) Cold pressed (i.e., unprocessed) vegetable oils should be used. These include linseed oil, cottonseed oil, safflower oil, soy oil, and peanut oil.

(10) Adults should drink 6 to 12 eight-ounce glasses of water daily depending upon body weight and climatic conditions. The best water to drink is distilled water because it has no carcinogenic agents or mineral excesses that are found in many water supplies. Also, there will be no chloride as there is in many city water supplies.

(11) Avoid caffeine in coffee, nonherb teas, and cola drinks. Caffeine is a stimulant that is addictive in most people. It can lead to glucose metabolism dysfunction.

(12) Alcohol is a refined carbohydrate, and like all refined carbohydrates, it should be avoided (except in cooking).

VITAMIN AND MINERAL SUPPLEMENTS

A diet of naturally produced natural foods would supply our bodies with the nutrients we need. But, unfortunately, because of our polluted air, water, and land, the growing of uncontaminated foods has become increasingly difficult, and by the time we see the foods in the market they have been further adulterated by all the processing and refining. Even fruits and vegetables are routinely subjected to artificial ripening by chemicals and coated with wax to prevent spoilage due to water evaporation. Dyes are also used to make the fruits and vegetables seem fresher and more appealing.

For these reasons, mineral and vitamin supplements are necessary to safeguard us against deficiencies and toxicities that cause the degenerative Killer Diseases.

We emphasize that we are not speaking here of therapeutic programs—each of which must be tailored to individual needs —but are making suggestions for vitamin and mineral supplements to accompany the general eating and lifestyle plan already set forth. (For additional important information, see appendixes B and C.)

Vitamin A. From 30,000 to 50,000 IU (international units) are recommended. Vitamin A is sometimes considered (along with vitamin D) to be one of the potentially toxic vitamins when taken in large amounts. However, in 15 years of medical practice, Dr. Harper has seen only three cases of toxicity due to vitamin A. In each of these cases it was due to drinking excessive amounts of carrot juice. He has treated patients with up to 200,000 IU a day without the toxic reactions of staining on the palm and inner foot areas, the turning of the whites of the eyes to a yellowish orange, nausea, diarrhea, dry, itchy and flaky skin, and/or hair loss.

Vitamin A is responsible for a great number of healthy tissues, including the hair and skin. Ironically, both a deficiency and an overdose result in dry, rough skin and loss of hair. Vitamin A is an excellent healing agent in burns and infections.

Vitamin B complex. This includes 11 vitamins whose functions are interrelated, so large doses of a few will cause deficiencies in the others. These vitamins are necessary for a wide range of metabolic responses including converting carbohydrates to glucose. They are necessary for the normal functioning of the nervous system and muscles, including the heart muscle, and are also necessary for healthy hair, skin, eyes, and mouth. Niacin (B_3) has been found useful in the treatment of schizophrenia and, along with B_6 and zinc, in the successful treatment of mentally affected patients.

Refining and cooking remove most B vitamins. "Enrichment" replaces only a few of them, usually B_1, B_2, and B_3. Additional amounts of B complex are needed during times of stress, when excessive amounts of alcohol are consumed and when there is a high consumption of refined carbohydrates.

Vitamin B_{15} and vitamin B_{17}. While not generally recognized in this country as vitamins per se, these substances are increasingly being demonstrated as useful metabolic agents and as effective in the prevention and management of cancer and other disease states. Despite the problems in this country with the availability of processed amygdalin (Laetrile), B_{17} is naturally abundant in the seeds of all fruits except citrus fruits and in large concentrations in apricot, peach, plum, and cherry seeds. It is also found in many grasses and several cereals. Vitamin B_{15}, or pangamic acid, is also found in many seeds as well as in rice hulls. We suggested in chapter four the generally good habit of consuming some peach or apricot kernels a day, not only because of their likely effect in preventing cancer, but because such seeds are laden with other important vitamins and minerals as well.

Vitamin C. Only two creatures within the mammalian kingdom are unable to produce vitamin C in their bodies: man and the guinea pig.

Vitamin C, or ascorbic acid, is a natural healing factor and there is evidence that it strengthens the body's first line of defense against disease. From 2,000 to 5,000 milligrams a day are recommended for all-around good health.

Chemist Irwin Stone, Nobel Prize winner Linus Pauling, and Dr. Ewan Cameron have led the fight for the recognition of megadoses of vitamin C for therapeutic use in fighting disease states that include cancer and the common cold. It has been an uphill fight, with the National Academy of Sciences even refusing to publish Pauling's vital biochemical studies on vitamin C. In addition, key findings of a Canadian study on the vitamin were at least partially suppressed. In this investigation, 5,000 Canadians were given daily doses of vitamin C at levels even under that which has been "generally recommended" by the research scientists. These people were matched against 5,000 in the general population who had not received the supplementary vitamin C. The result was that absenteeism for *all* kinds of disease was lower for the group taking the small amount of supplemental vitamin C.

Vitamin D. Vitamin D is something of a problem because there can be too much of it in the body. There are 27 different agents available that are called vitamin D, but only sunlight and fish liver oil are sources of the type of vitamin D necessary to man—that is, vitamin D_3. Adequate quantities of vitamin D_3 are normally produced in the body by the exposure of the mellanin cells of the skin to sunshine. No supplements are needed, though additional vitamin D_3 may be absorbed by taking fish liver oil.

The vitamin D that is said to "enrich" or "fortify" milk and other foods is actually vitamin D_2, or irradiated ergosterol, a plant steroid derived from exposing plants to ultraviolet light. Vitamin D_2, was outlawed in Germany over 50 years ago because of its link to calcification in the heart valves of children. Vitamin D_2 also causes the demineralization of bones and may contribute to the deposit of calcium in abnormal locations such as in the joints and in arteriosclerotic plaques.

Vitamin E. Controversy over vitamin E has raged since its discovery earlier this century, and only now is it becoming accepted as an effective antioxidant and anticoagulant and as a healing agent. It helps prevent heart disease, slows down the aging process, and exhibits a general benign metabolic effect throughout the body. It also protects the cell membranes from the free radicals of "unbonded" minerals such as lead and excessive calcium, which adversely affect the cell membrane wall. For this reason it is referred to as a free radical scavenger.

Vitamin E helps to decrease "blood-platelet agglutination," which is the congealing within arteries of platelets in the bloodstream, a process that is enhanced by the continual ingestion of sugar which causes an increased "stickiness" of the platelets. Unfortunately, orthodoxy is relying on aspirin to decrease platelet agglutination, but bleeding ulcers and increased stomach acidity are the risks of continual aspirin use. On the other hand, side effects are extremely rare from vitamin E, except for causing elevated blood pressure in some people, especially hypertensives, who should have their blood pressure checked within a week of adding vitamin E to their diet.

D-alpha tocopherol succinate is the better, more potent form of vitamin E because it is absorbed better than the d-alpha tocopherol acetate, which is an oil-based solution, as compared to the water-based solution of the succinate. The alpha tocopherol is also superior to the mixed tocopherols. A daily supplement of 200 IU of the succinate form or 400 IU of the acetate form is recommended.

Minerals. An adequate supply of trace minerals should be taken as part of normal nutrition because they furnish the atoms from which the molecules of enzymes—those body catalysts which cause chemical changes—are made. Each of the 5,300 known enzyme systems in the body is activated by trace minerals. Too many or too few of any of these minerals can cause severe metabolic disorders.

Magnesium. The mineral most commonly in short supply in man is magnesium, which activates 80 percent of the body's enzyme systems. A deficiency may lead to a number of disease states, the most severe being magnesium deficiency psychosis, which mimics catatonic schizophrenia. A determination of the exact needs of each individual can be made through a hair analysis (see pages 78–79).

Magnesium is in all the foods listed under it in appendix C, but if taken in tablet form it should be administered as an amino acid compound. A common magnesium supplement is dolomite, a combination of calcium and magnesium that has been known to contain particles of lead. Magnesium complexed with orotatic acid as magnesium orotate makes an excellent tablet source. Either the natural food sources or tablets taken three times a day should supply the body with adequate magnesium.

Manganese. This is a necessary mineral that is used by various enzyme systems and that, with magnesium, is responsible for balancing the autonomic nervous system that controls automatic functions throughout the body. Manganese is involved in stimulating the activity of that system and magnesium is involved in suppressing it, so a correct balance is necessary for a balanced autonomic nervous system. The effects of both manganese and magnesium are influenced by calcium.

191

When supplementation of manganese is necessary, an amino acid–manganese complex gives the best results.

Magnesium, calcium, and manganese compete for absorption in the small intestine, and therefore when they are taken at the same time, they are not absorbed well. When a deficiency in more than one of these minerals is involved, they are best taken separately with four or more hours' difference in the time of ingestion. Manganese is best given in the morning since it has a stimulating effect on the autonomic nervous system, and magnesium should be taken at bedtime since it has a depressing effect upon that system and may cause drowsiness. Calcium can be taken during the middle of the day if it is necessary.

Calcium. The problem with calcium is apt to be too much rather than too little—or at least too much in the wrong places—since in the American diet calcium is obtained in large quantities of milk and milk products. Ironically, there may be too much calcium where it is not needed and too little at the intracellular level. This cellular deficiency in calcium may affect normal heart tissue as well as other organic systems. The amino acid–calcium combination tablet, calcium orotate, taken three times a day for a total of about 750 mg a day, is a sound way to compensate for calcium deficiency when it does occur.

Many people, especially our "senior citizens," have been misguided and led to take bone meal for their calcium deficiencies. This product is obtained by grinding up the bones of animals, but there is a risk here. The animals whose bones are used in the process have consumed large amounts of grazing grasses and grains in which have been deposited toxic chemicals from industrial pollution, including lead, for which the body has no need and which is toxic to man. This lead may be deposited in the red blood cells and bones of the animals which are later slaughtered, but slaughtering does not diminish the lead content in the bones. Bone meal should be avoided as a supplement inasmuch as lead levels up to 28 parts per million have been found in it.

Zinc and chromium. These two minerals are, among other things, used in the production of insulin by the pancreas and are thus highly important in terms of controlling blood sugar levels. Feeding test animals diets deficient in zinc has produced diabetes in them. An atom of zinc is present in every molecule of insulin. Chromium is another of the "two-edged sword" minerals. It is used in the conversion of pro-insulin into insulin and is needed in small quantities in the body. However, chromium toxicity can occur with too much intake of the mineral, which can result because of the fact that it is used as an anticorrosive agent in the air conditioning industry. Chromium may be deposited in the lungs and kidneys. There is a high correlation between hexavalent chromium and cancer in test animals.

The polluting of an industrial population by the hexavalent form of chromium should have made headlines in 1976 when the material, used in the factory cooling system of a well known electronics firm, mixed in with the factory drinking water after a valve malfunctioned. The yellowishness and peculiar taste of the contaminated water was noticed by one of the 91 employees, who alerted the management. Samples of the blood of 20 of the 91 workers were subjected to mineral analysis and chromium contamination was found in all 20. Since not only was the chromium toxicity probably in all 91 workers, but also in other people who entered the building from time to time, a lengthy program to trace and treat the contaminated was discussed, but the information was suppressed since it was determined that the entire program might cost as much as $6 million. Batteries of medical researchers were called in for their points of view until a residue could be found of those experts who decided that no major problem had occurred because of the chromium contamination. It will take years to determine whether the contaminated people develop disproportionate amounts of leukemia and/or cancer of the kidneys and lungs.

Zinc is also vital to the body's healing mechanism and is active against infections and skin lesions.

Copper. This is another mineral in which the problem is more likely to be too much rather than too little in our society because of the prevalence of copper piping in homes and apartments. Acidification may result in increased copper concentration in the water. Excessive amounts of the mineral may affect the central nervous system and cause depression and other psychological problems.

Sodium and potassium. These are the "transporters" of the cellular system, and they bring needed minerals across the cell membrane into the cell itself. While there is rarely a deficiency in sodium because of our love of salt, excessive sodium has been linked to congestive heart failure.

Potassium deficiencies show up in a number of disease states and frequently occur as a result of a "doctor-caused," or iatrogenic, treatment, especially the overadministration of diuretics, or "water pills." Excessive potassium levels may induce ulcerative lesions in the intestines, so potassium tablets should only be taken after meals or as a liquid.

Lead, cadmium, and mercury. These are toxic minerals for which the body has no known use and any amount is regarded as excessive.

We have already pointed to lead, particularly from gasoline, as a major atmospheric and food polluter. In fact, one of the easiest ways to build up lead toxicity is to be seated in an automobile idling at a stoplight. A defective muffler, manifold, or exhaust system will spew the exhaust fumes into the car. It may also enter the body from certain hair dyes. Lead poisoning affects the whole body, particularly the nervous system, and takes the place of "lighter" minerals in the body that are needed by the enzyme systems.

Cadmium causes high blood pressure and other negative conditions and is taken into the body from cigarette smoke as well as from industrial pollution.

The worst effects of mercury are on the nervous system. It is most likely to be ingested by eating fish that were caught in shallow, polluted waters or that routinely feed on bottom fish from lakes, ponds, and streams polluted by mercury from industrial waste. There is a growing suspicion that mercury, a principal ingredient of the amalgam used to fill cavities, may correlate with the unusually high suicide rate among dentists and dental assistants who mix the amalgam and thereby contaminate themselves.

SIX

For Freedom of Choice and Informed Consent

In the past decade there has been a clamor over the "right to die"—a patient's right to expire when all existing treatments for his condition have been tried and have failed and he does not wish to be kept alive by means of some form of gadgetry.

Ironically, there has been less concern over what might be called the patient's "right to live." But if there is a single message we would like to give, it is that this right should be emphasized above all others.

In the modern world of manmade Killer Diseases that are decimating our population, patients are routinely being denied access to vital information that might very well save their lives and/or reduce their suffering. They are not aware that there are *alternatives* to slow death and surgical approaches to heart disease and that there are nontoxic, nutritional, nonsurgical treatments available for cancer.

Most physicians do not deliberately mislead their patients. They themselves have been misinformed or misled by the blind, arrogant, economically oriented, close-minded group consisting of the pharmaceutical-medical-technological-government "club."

The misinformed individual physician may also be swayed by his own vested interest either consciously or subconsciously. Let's face it: basic metabolic and nutritional approaches to the Killer Diseases, including the use of chelation therapy in heart disease, pose relatively inexpensive solutions to 80 percent of the nation's total health problem. And, of course, prevention itself stands to wipe out this huge factor in the health-care delivery industry and the legion of specialists, internists, diagnosticians, clinics, hospitals, insurance, technological software, expensive drugs, and surgical experts that goes with it.

Patients *must* be given the opportunity for a truly informed consent. In cardiovascular surgery, for example, they *must* be told what the mortality rates for the operation they are being offered really are. These facts and figures must not be covered up by mellifluous euphemisms. The patients must not be rushed into operations through high-pressure scare tactics employed upon them and their families.

Patients must also be told of nutritional and metabolic alternatives to standard treatment. However, they cannot be told about them if their attending physicians know nothing about them. And the physicians will know nothing about them as long as a small elite is in control of the nation's medical schools and research facilities and is also in control of funds for research and propaganda.

The tendency of the uninformed physician is to reject something he does not know about. Thus his judgment on, say, chelation therapy, will be based on a *lack* of evidence, rather than on objective observation. How can a physician make a judgment on a therapeutic program if he has not seen how it works? Only those with personal experience either as a physician or a patient will be able to make objective judgments.

Unfortunately, metabolic, or nutritional, therapists are usually the last doctors to whom patients turn after they have been rotated through the turnstiles of orthodox medicine, whose approaches and nostrums have failed. Hence, the metabolic or nutritional therapist is apt to be seeing, a majority of the time, only those who are desperate and whose chances for survival or meaningful alleviation are minimal at best.

It is grossly unjust that physicians who specialize in metabolic and nutritional therapy and preventive medicine are victims of peer-group pressure through medical licensing boards controlled by the representatives of a single school of medicine. It is a national disgrace that they should sometimes actually be open to arrest, fines, and even imprisonment for making available alternative therapies to victims of the Killer Diseases and being faithful to their Hippocratic Oath to treat patients to the best of their ability.

American citizens should have the right to freedom of

choice in therapy—that is, the right to opt for therapies based on the informed consent of themselves and their physicians. It is outrageous that the federal government and state boards of medicine should in any way interfere with the sacred physician-patient relationship.

It is disturbing that there exists a comfortable relationship between the purveyors of food pollution, the peddlers of drugs to "cure" us of and/or to mask the symptoms of such pollution, and the federal regulatory agencies that supposedly were created to act on behalf of the citizen.

The answer to breaking the economic domination of the drug cartel and the misleading advertising and propaganda of the major food processors is not to be found so much in building yet more governmental control—for giant government and giant monopolies only become each other's tools—but in the restoration of a truly free market in these industries. This implies economic solutions that can only be imposed through political awareness.

There must also be a free marketplace of ideas in the monopolistic, one-sided world of American medicine. The utter lack of nutritional education among physicians is appalling and is at the root of most of our medical distress. But this lack will not be corrected until an informed public and more physicians themselves rise up in anger and demand it.

The ultimate challenge in ending the needless slaughter of the Killer Diseases is to marshal the strongest force in a free society—an informed public—so that necessary change can take place.

The Harper Eating Plan for Glucose Metabolism Dysfunction

THE BASIC PLAN

BASIC RULES

(1) You will have small frequent feedings. *Eat at least every 2½ hours or more during your waking hours.*

(2) You will eat *protein foods, vegetables, and fruits.* All refined carbohydrates (sugar and flour) will be eliminated. If you are overweight, most fats will also be eliminated.

(3) You will supplement your food with a protein drink.

(4) You will take vitamin and mineral supplements.

PROTEIN FOODS

Eat allowed protein foods at least *four* times each day. For the first 3 months eat protein every 2½ hours. Each feeding should include at least a small piece of fruit or vegetable plus 1 ounce of cheese, or 2 ounces of meat, poultry or seafood, or 3 ounces of cottage cheese, or 1 cup of yogurt. After the first three to six months, you may have protein only *four* times each day with fruits and vegetables as snacks. You *must* eat at least 3 ounces of protein for breakfast.

Eat at least 16 ounces of protein each day. For overweight, no more than 16 ounces each day.

Problem sleepers: eat 4 ounces of protein before bedtime.

Not Allowed

Milk of any kind. It contains lactose, a rapidly metabolized sugar.

Processed meat or cheese

Beans (except green and wax)

Not Allowed for Overweight, Otherwise Allowed

Butter

Cream

Cream cheese

Fatty meats

Jones brand sausage

Nuts and seeds. Purchase raw only. No more than 2 to 3 ounces each day.

Oil-packed fish

Sour cream

Yogurt (Never use preflavored yogurt.)

Allowed

All meats, poultry (without skin), seafood, except those packaged with sugar or preservatives.

Eggs. No more than 7 per week for overweight. Each egg counts as 2 ounces of protein.

White cheeses. No more than 2 or 4 ounces each day. For overweight, no more than 1 ounce per day.

Low-fat cottage cheese. No more than 4 ounces each day for overweight.

Ham and other cured meats. Not allowed for severe hypoglycemia or diabetes. Limit to 2 ounces per day when tolerated.

Canadian bacon. Not allowed for severe hypoglycemia or diabetes.

Armour Micra-Cure bacon. Limit to 3 slices per day.

VEGETABLES

Eat at least 2 to 4 cups of vegetables each day.

Use raw salad vegetables freely.

Use only 1 "limited" vegetable each day (or not at all). No more than ½ cup per serving.

Leafy green and stalk vegetables are best.

Not Allowed

Corn
Jerusalem artichokes
Peas
Potatoes
Rice
Starchy beans

Allowed in Limited Quantities

Acorn and butternut squash
Beets and beet juice
Carrots and carrot juice
Globe artichokes
Onions. May be used freely in cooking.
Parsnips

Allowed

All other vegetables.
Tomato juice and V-8 juice count as vegetables. Up to 16 oz. each day.

FRUITS

No more than 3 servings of fruit each day are allowed.
Each serving is the size of one medium apple.
Never have more than one fruit serving per feeding.
For overweight limit fruit to 2 servings each day.

Not Allowed

Apple juice
Bananas
Dried fruit
Grapes
Grape juice
Prune juice
Sweetened canned fruit
Watermelon

Allowed in Limited Quantities

Avocados. Not allowed for overweight. Otherwise no more than ½ avocado per serving.

Cherries. No more than 6 per serving.

Mangos. No more than one mango per week, no more than ½ per serving.

Persimmons. No more than one medium persimmon per week.

All fruit juices except those listed as "not allowed." About 4 ounces of juice equal one serving of fruit.

Allowed

All other fruits. Melons and berries are best.

FATS

Not Allowed for Overweight

All fats and oils are not allowed except for *occasional* use of nonhydrogenated vegetable oils.

No butter, margarine, lard, or fatty meats.

You may use Pam and other similar products.

Allowed for Normal and Underweight

Cold pressed vegetable oils such as safflower, soy, peanut, and sesame.

Margarine made from safflower oil.

GRAINS

Not Allowed

All grains, whole or refined, except wheat germ and raw, unprocessed bran. You may have up to 2 tablespoons of wheat germ and 2 tablespoons of bran each day.

Any product made from grains such as flour, cereals and pasta.

No bread of any kind made with flour or processed grain.

OTHER FOODS NOT ALLOWED

Carbohydrates

Carbohydrates are *not* allowed, except those found in allowed foods.

No sweeteners of any kind except artificial.
Severe hypoglycemics may react to sorbitol and manitol.

Caffeine

No caffeine is allowed. This includes coffee, tea, cola drinks, Dr. Pepper, Mountain Dew, or painkillers with caffeine.

Alcoholic Beverages

No alcoholic beverages are allowed.
Wine may be used in cooking.

THE PROTEIN DRINK

Have a Protein Drink

(1) Upon arising in the morning.
(2) One-half hour prior to your afternoon low.
(3) ANYTIME you feel low or cranky.

Make the Protein Drink with

1 heaping tablespoon protein powder
1 teaspoon brewer's yeast flakes
4 ounces (½ cup) liquid
1–4 ice cubes (optional)
Place ingredients in a blender and mix well.

Use a protein powder that is *90 percent protein or more with no carbohydrates*.

The liquid to use is any flavored diet soda, orange juice, grapefruit juice, or tomato juice. Orange or grapefruit juice counts as a fruit.

VITAMINS AND MINERALS

Hypoglycemics and diabetics should have a hair analysis to check for mineral imbalances.

The following vitamins and minerals are basic. Additions may be made on an individual basis.

Vitamin E

Take 400 IU each day. Use d-alpha tocopherol rather than mixed tocopherol.

B Complex with C

Take 2 capsules twice each day of the following formula:

Thiamin mononitrate (B1) . . . . .15 mg
Riboflavin (B2) . . . . .10 mg
Pyridoxine HCL (B6) . . . . .5 mg
Nicotinamine (or niacinamide) . . . . .50 mg
Calcium pantothenate . . . . .10 mg
Ascorbic acid (vitamin C) . . . . .300 mg

Amino Acid Tablets

Use a multiple amino acid plus minerals. Take as directed on label. Suitable brands are Minamino, Amino/Min, AG/Pro, or Uni-Pro 9. With Uni-Pro 9 a mineral supplement is necessary.

MISCELLANEOUS

Drink at least 2 quarts of spring, distilled, or filtered water each day. This acts as a natural laxative and prevents kidney stones.

Stop smoking or at least cut down to 5 to 10 cigarettes a day. Use the protein drink to satisfy cravings.

Use a small postage scale for measuring your protein.

Excellent recipes for this Eating Plan can be found in *The Low Blood Sugar Cookbook* by Marie Blevin and Geri Ginder (Doubleday) or in either of the *Dr. Atkins' Diet Revolution* books.

Read all labels. Avoid all sugars and starches.

THE EXTENDED EATING PLAN

After you have been on the Harper Eating Plan for Glucose Metabolism Dysfunction for at least three months, and after you have had *one symptom-free month* (see the Health Indicator Test, pages 62–63), you may start adding certain foods. The following list of foods is very general and must be approached with caution.

Select *one* food item at a time to add to the basic Eating Plan. Wait at least *two days* to see if you have a reaction. If there is none, i.e. you have no loss of energy, you do not get a headache, and you do not become irritable or depressed, then you may continue that food in limited quantities. Because you do not have a reaction to a certain food does not mean you may indulge in that food. Moderation should always prevail.

PROTEIN FOODS

You may now cut your protein intake down to 10 ounces each day.

Protein should still be eaten at least 4 times daily and you must continue your snacks.

Foods to Add

Nonfat dry milk. This can be used for "breading" and in cooking.
Low-fat milk. Preferably raw. No more than 4 ounces per day.
Soy beans, cooked or roasted. Two to four ounces per day.
Soy flour. Use for bread and in recipes calling for flour. No more than two slices of bread per day.
Gluten flour. Use the same as soy flour.

VEGETABLES

You may have one serving of only one of these vegetables per week.

Always eat these vegetables along with 4 to 6 ounces of protein.

Add

Corn. No more than ½ cup per serving.
Unpolished brown rice. Two to four ounces cooked weight.
Wild rice. Two to four ounces cooked weight. No polished or refined rice.
Potatoes. Baked only, with the skin. Start by scooping out most of the potato and eating the skin and a small layer of potato. You may work up to a medium baked potato.

FRUITS

Add

Watermelon. One-half of an average slice one inch thick. No more than once a week.

GRAINS

Add

Whole grains. You may make your own granola with whole grains. Be careful if you buy prepared granola as many brands contain brown sugar, honey, raisins, or dates.

Whole grain bread. Many markets and most health food stores carry a seven-grain 100 percent stone-ground bread. Use only one slice per day and always with 2 to 4 ounces of protein.

Oat flour and old-fashioned rolled oats. No more than ½ cup cooked oats per serving. Use oat flour for bread and recipes calling for flour.

ALCOHOLIC BEVERAGES

If you are an alcoholic or have any kind of drinking problem, forget about ever adding alcohol to the Eating Plan. It is not worth the aggravation that can result.

Other hypoglycemics must stay away from all alcohol until one symptom-free month has passed. After that time you may have an *occasional* drink. Watch your reactions very carefully.

Always drink distilled spirits such as vodka, tequila, gin, bourbon, and scotch, or dry wine. Always mix the liquor with water, diet soda, or club soda—*it must be diluted*. Do not drink unless you have a few ounces of protein along with it. You may not have any more than one or two drinks a day, no more than two days per week.

A Guide to Vitamins and Minerals

Nutrient	Functions	Adult RDA	Optimum Metabolic Supplementation Recommendations for "Healthy" People	Deficiency Symptoms	Toxicity Symptoms	Comments
Vitamin A	Fights infections Helps repair body tissues Induces healthy hair and a good complexion Involved in the digestion of proteins Reduces cholesterol Helps in the prevention and treatment of cancer	5,000 IU	30,000–50,000 IU	Increased susceptibility to infections Dry, scaly skin Lack of appetite Night blindness Fatigue	Nausea, diarrhea Dry, itchy skin Staining on palms of hands and soles of feet Whites of eyes turn yellowish orange	Absorption hindered by alcohol, iron, cortisone, mineral oil Absorption hindered by physical exercise within four hours of ingestion Excessive loss of vitamin A may occur when one has cancer, tuberculosis, or infections
Vitamin B1 (thiamine)	Carbohydrate metabolism	0.5 mg per 1000 calories	50–150 mg	Loss of appetite Digestive disturbances	None known	Required when on long-term thyroid replacement therapy
Vitamin B2 (riboflavin)	Involved in digestion of proteins, fats, and carbohydrates Necessary for healthy eyes and good vision Aids in absorption of iron	Males: 1.6 mg Females: 1.2 mg	30–100 mg	Digestive disturbances Problems with sight Mouth sores Dermatitis	None known	Animal experiments show cancer is inhibited

Nutrient	Functions	Adult RDA	Supplementation Recommendations for "Healthy" People	Deficiency Symptoms	Toxicity Symptoms	Comments
Vitamin B15 (pangamic acid)	Increases oxygen supply to cells Necessary for proper functioning of nervous system and glandular system Involved in digestion of proteins Involved in glucose regulation	Not established	100–200 mg	Nervous system disorders Insufficient oxygen to cells	None known	Widely used in Russia, where many clinical tests have been performed to establish its need in human nutrition
Vitamin B17 (Laetrile)	Prevents and helps in the treatment of cancer Decreases pain in terminal cancer patients Increases appetite in cancer patients Decreases or eliminates metastasis (spread) of cancer cells Regulates blood pressure	Not established	100–500 mg	May result in cancer	None known	Not approved for use in United States by FDA, which claims it may be poisonous due to the cyanide it contains Advocates claim the cyanide is detoxified in normal cells by enzyme called rhodanese, which is not in cancer cells and thus Laetrile attacks only these cancer cells Present in 1,400 natural, unrefined foods
Vitamin B3 (niacin)	Involved in digestion of proteins, fats, and carbohydrates Necessary for proper functioning of nervous system Necessary for proper functioning of digestive system Improves circulation Reduces cholesterol and triglycerides	Males: 18 mg Females: 13 mg	200–400 mg	Dermatitis Nervous system disorders Fatigue Loss of appetite Insomnia Headaches Irritability	None known, but may cause flushing and/or tingling or itching due to dilation of capillaries in surface of skin	Used in combination with B6 and zinc in high dosage levels in treatment of schizophrenia Antibiotics and refined carbohydrates cause excessive loss of niacin May prevent cancer due to enzyme regulation
Vitamin B6 (pyrodoxine)	Involved in digestion of proteins, fats, and carbohydrates Necessary for proper functioning of nervous system Necessary for production of antibodies by body Required for proper absorption of B12 and magnesium Necessary for proper balance of sodium and potassium	2 mg per 100 grams protein per day	50–200 mg	Anemia Glucose metabolism dysfunction Hair loss Arthritis Nervousness Depression Irritability Increased urination	None known	Treatment for arthritis involves use of vitamin B6 in dosages as high as 300–600 mg daily Used in treatment of heart failure

Optimum Metabolic Supplementation Recommendations for "Healthy" People

Nutrient	Functions	Adult RDA	Optimum Metabolic Supplementation Recommendations for "Healthy" People	Deficiency Symptoms	Toxicity Symptoms	Comments
Vitamin B12	Involved in digestion of proteins, fats, and carbohydrates. Necessary for metabolism of nerve tissue	3 mcg	200–1,000 mcg	Anemia Fatigue Nervousness Irritability Inability to concentrate Depression Insomnia	None known	Calcium is needed with vitamin B12 for proper absorption by body Vegetarians develop deficiencies easily Only vitamin that contains essential mineral elements Produced in stomach with intrinsic factor; deficiencies commonly occur after stomach surgery
Biotin (a B complex vitamin)	Involved in digestion of proteins, fats, and carbohydrates. Necessary for body to utilize folic acid, B12, and pantothenic acid	Not established	300–600 mcg	Muscle pain Loss of appetite Lack of energy Dry skin Insomnia Depression	None known	Trace amounts appear in all animal and plant tissue
Choline (a B complex vitamin)	Involved in digestion and transportation of fats. Essential for health of liver and kidney. Necessary for protection of myelin sheath of nerves	Not established	1,000–2,000 mg	Ulcers Hemorrhaging of kidneys High blood pressure	None known	**Overdosage may cause deficiency in B6** Aids in prevention of gallstones
Folic acid (a B complex vitamin)	Involved in metabolism of proteins. Involved in red blood cell formation	400 mcg	400–1,000 mcg	Anemia Digestive disorders	None known	**Large amounts should be administered only under directions of a physician**
Inositol (a B complex vitamin)	Necessary for formation of lecithin. Involved in metabolism of fats	Not established	500–1,000 mg	Loss of hair Constipation High cholesterol	None known	Caffeine may cause deficiency Protects liver, kidney and heart Helps reduce cholesterol
PABA (para-aminobenzoic acid; a B complex vitamin)	Involved in digestion and utilization of proteins. Involved in formation of red blood cells. Necessary for healthy skin	Not established	100–300 mg	Digestive disorders Fatigue Depression Irritability Headaches Nervousness	Nausea, vomiting	Sulfa drugs cause deficiency
Pantothenic acid (calcium	Involved in release of energy from proteins, fats and car-	5–10 mg estimated to be ade-	20–50 mg	Digestive disorders Restlessness	None known	Stimulates adrenal glands Aids body in withstanding

Vitamin	Functions	Recommended Daily Allowance	Deficiency Symptoms	Comments
Vitamin C (ascorbic acid)	Maintains collagen (a protein that binds all our cells and bones) Strengthens capillary walls Fights infections Necessary for healthy skin Aids in healing Necessary for metabolism of amino acids Aids in utilization of iron Helps in the prevention and treatment of cancer	Males: 60 mg Females: 55 mg	2,000–5,000 mg	Digestive disorders Slow healing time Bruising Bleeding gums Shortness of breath	None known	**Take in several small dosages during day rather than in one large dose** Take vitamin C with iron as it aids body in absorbing iron Increase dosage when fighting infection May ease pain in arthritic patients by thinning lubricating fluid of joints making movement of these joints easier Believed to protect man against cancer-causing nitrates and nitrites Decreases incidence of viral infections; large doses of 10,000 to 100,000 mg daily used in treatment of viral infections

Nutrient	Functions	Adult RDA	Optimum Metabolic Supplementation Recommendations for "Healthy" People	Deficiency Symptoms	Toxicity Symptoms	Comments
Vitamin D	Aids in absorption of calcium Aids in metabolism of phosphorus which is necessary for bone formation	400 IU	15 to 30 minutes in sunlight or 1 tablespoon of cod liver oil 400 IU from natural fish liver oil	Soft bones Irritability Tetany	Calcification of walls of blood vessels and demineralization of bone is caused by D2 (a plant steroid)	**Vitamin D2, the form most often found in supplements and which is said to "fortify" milk in the United States, should be avoided as it causes calcification of heart valves and other tissues** Vitamin D3 is nontoxic and most people get sufficient amount through exposure to sunlight; fish liver oil is only other natural source of D3
Vitamin E	Promotes healing and retards scarring Protects red blood cells Strengthens capillary walls	15 IU	200–800 IU	Angina Intermittent claudication	None, with the exception of raising blood pressure in some people	**Hypertensives should have blood pressure checked one week after adding to diet** **Do not take at same time as iron or hormones**

Nutrient	Function		Deficiency Symptoms	Overdose Symptoms	Comments
	Acts as antioxidant Dilates blood vessels which results in better circulation Helps in the prevention and treatment of cancer				Take before meals Take d-alpha tocopherol succinate as it is absorbed more easily and therefore this is the most potent and gives the greatest benefits
Vitamin K	Involved in formation of prothrombin which is necessary for blood to clot	Not established	None	Hemorrhaging Diarrhea Nosebleeds	None with natural vitamin K Flushing, sweating, constriction of chest with synthetic vitamin K	Adequate amounts of vitamin K are normally produced in the intestinal tract except in cases of long-term ingestion or oral antibodies. Yogurt, buttermilk or acidophilus milk should be included in the diet to help the body establish normal intestinal flora to manufacture vitamin K when antibiotics are taken
Cadmium	None—toxic mineral that has no function in human body	None	None	May cause hypertension Muscle weakness Nervous system functions may be affected	Found primarily in refined foods and in air as industrial pollutant Also in coffee, tea, and tobacco Zinc keeps toxicity of cadmium in check

Nutrient	Functions	Adult RDA	Optimum Metabolic Supplementation Recommendations for "Healthy" People	Deficiency Symptoms	Toxicity Symptoms	Comments
Calcium	Assists in normal blood clotting Involved in muscle growth and contraction Necessary for normal heart function Involved in normal nerve transmission Aids in utilization of iron	800 mg	250–1,000 mg as calcium oratate	Tetany Muscle cramps Insomnia Irritability	Calcification of soft tissues	Must be taken with magnesium, phosphorus and vitamins A and C to function properly in body. **In a deficiency state of the body, calcium should not be taken orally at the same time as magnesium or manganese, since these minerals compete with calcium for absorption in the intestinal tract**
Chromium	Involved in metabolism of glucose Helps regulate blood sugar levels	Not established	500–1,000 mcg divalent (2+ charge) chromium	Glucose metabolism dysfunction	Hexavalent (6+ charge) chromium is a strong carcinogenic agent and may cause cancer of lungs and kidneys	Hexavalent chromium is not traceable in bloodstream 72 hours after exposure since it is deposited in kidney and lung tissue; traceable from deposits in hair and nails for extended time after exposure

Mineral	Functions	Dosage	Deficiency symptoms	Toxicity symptoms	Notes
Copper	Aids in formation of red blood cells Involved in metabolism of amino acids Involved in healing	2 mg	2 mg, complexed with amino acids	Weakness Skin sores Difficulty in breathing	Mental retardation Hyperactivity Depression Hypertension Arteriosclerosis	Deposited in excess in Wilson's disease (an inherited disease) in liver, eyes, and central nervous system and can cause mental retardation and even death if not removed from body. Chelating agents such as BAL and penicillamine used to remove excesses from the body Metabolized through liver and other tissue
Iodine	Aids in functioning of thyroid gland Involved in regulation of body's energy Involved in regulating rate of metabolism Necessary for healthy nails, skin, hair, and teeth	Males: 130 mcg Females: 100 mcg	100–300 mcg	Hypothyroidism Obesity Slowed mental reactions Nervousness Irritability Cretinism (dwarfism with mental retardation) Thyroid cysts, or goiters	Rapid pulse	Toxicity is rare

Nutrient	Functions	Adult RDA	Optimum Metabolic Supplementation Recommendations for "Healthy" People	Deficiency Symptoms	Toxicity Symptoms	Comments
Iron	Necessary for formation of hemoglobin. Necessary for formation of myoglobin. Increases resistance to disease and stress. Involved in protein metabolism	Males: 10 mg Females: 18 mg	20–50 mg	Anemia. Abnormal fatigue. Malfunction of central nervous system and transmission of nerve impulses	Hemosiderosis (excess iron). Dizziness. Loss of weight. Headache. Shortness of breath. Fatigue	Excess deposits of iron affect liver, lungs, pancreas and heart
Lead	None	None	None	None	Colic. Anemia. Brain dysfunction. Hyperactivity. Mental retardation. Fatigue. Convulsions	Chief source of lead is auto emissions; 30,000 pounds of lead are discharged daily from auto exhaust in the Los Angeles basin alone. Lead toxicity also comes from cigarettes, burning coal, and lead-based paints
Magnesium	Activates enzymes necessary for metabolism of amino acids and carbohydrates	Males: 350 mg Females: 300 mg	350–1,000 mg as magnesium orotate	Tremors. Confusion. Anxiety. Heart disease	Depression of central nervous system	**Do not take after meals** Very common mineral deficiency; needed in most enzyme systems. Toxicity is rare

Mineral	Function	Recommended amount	Amount in body	Deficiency symptoms	Toxicity symptoms	Comments
	Involved in proper functioning of muscles and nerves Necessary for metabolism and absorption of calcium, sodium, phosphorus, and potassium					Most common mineral deficiency
Manganese	Used in various enzyme systems Stimulates the activity of the automatic functions of the nervous system	Not established	5–20 mg complexed with amino acids	Glucose metabolism dysfunction Dizziness Loss of hearing Convulsions	Storage of iron Irritability Tremor Muscle rigidity	
Mercury	None	None		None	Psychosis Blindness Paralysis Convulsions Kidney damage	Sources are industrial pollution, fish, burning coal

Nutrient	Functions	Adult RDA	Optimum Metabolic Supplementation Recommendations for "Healthy" People	Deficiency Symptoms	Toxicity Symptoms	Comments
Phosphorus	Involved in utilization of proteins, fats, and carbohydrates for tissue growth and repair and for production of energy Necessary for proper functioning of nervous system Necessary for proper functioning of kidneys	800 mg	Rarely needed as supplement; adequate amount in diet	Loss of appetite Fatigue Nervous disorders	None	Adequate amounts of phosphorus are normally available in the diet without additional supplements Serum calcium/phosphorus ratio should be 2.5/1 for optimum health; phosphorus level rises with ingestion of refined carbohydrates
Potassium	Necessary for proper distribution of fluids within body Involved in proper functioning of muscles and nerves Stimulates kidneys to eliminate toxic wastes Involved in cell metabolism and enzyme reactions	Not established	500–1,000 mg	Weakness Poor muscle tone Acne Dry skin Insomnia Nervous disorders Mental apathy Fatigue Constipation	None; rapidly excreted through kidneys when there is an excess	**Take after meals to avoid irritation of stomach** Deficiency occurs most often in patients taking diuretics (water pills), cortisone drugs, ACTH, digitalis and in patients with diabetes, high blood pressure, or liver disease Fruits and vegetables grown on soil lacking in potash have less natural potassium content

Selenium	Delays oxidation of polyunsaturated fatty acids Promotes normal body growth and fertility	Minuscule	50 mcg	Loss of tissue elasticity Loss of integrity of cellular membranes	Loss of hair, nails, and teeth Dermatitis Lassitude Progressive paralysis	**Selenium should be obtained only from diet as it can be toxic in its pure form** Works with vitamin E
Sodium	Involved in regulation of fluids within body Involved in proper functioning of muscles and nerves Removes carbon dioxide from body	Not established	None	Weight loss Vomiting Muscle shrinkage	Potassium deficiency	Sufficient sodium (and, in some cases, too much sodium) is obtained from table salt

Nutrient	Functions	Adult RDA	Optimum Metabolic Supplementation Recommendations for "Healthy" People	Deficiency Symptoms	Toxicity Symptoms	Comments
Zinc	Involved in absorption and actions of vitamins As component of enzymes, involved in digestion and metabolism Involved in carbohydrate digestion Involved in metabolism of phosphorus Involved in development of reproductive organs Necessary for proper functioning of prostate gland	15 mg	10–30 mg complexed with amino acids	Sterility Retarded growth Fatigue Loss of appetite Retarded wound healing Joint pain Birth defects Dwarfism Male growth lag Impotency in young males Menstrual aberrations Loss of taste and smell Glucose metabolism dysfunction	None	The percent of zinc in fruits and vegetables varies depending upon the zinc content of the soil. Nonrotation of crops causes continual depletion of the soil and artificial fertilizers do not usually contain zinc

High Mineral-Content Foods

FOODS HIGH IN CALCIUM

Green leaf and green stalk
   vegetables
Mustard greens
Turnip greens
Egg yolk
Milk and dairy products

Canned sardines and salmon
Shellfish
Broccoli
Kale
Soybeans

FOODS HIGH IN COPPER

American cheese
Sweet potatoes
Dried prunes
Citrus fruits
Beef liver
Pork chops
Mushrooms
Mackerel
Whole rye
Asparagus
Almonds
Avocados
Cabbage
Chicken
Beef
Kale

Lobster
Halibut
Grapes
Oats
Pecans
Oysters
Shrimp
Spinach
Turkey
Walnuts
Wheat
Eggs
Apples
Corn
Carrots

FOODS HIGH IN IRON

Dry apricots
Wheat germ

Liver sausage
All legumes

Soy beans
Lean meats
Egg yolk
Green leafy vegetables
Unprocessed whole grain
  cereals
Dry brewer's yeast

Liver
Peaches
Heart
Kidney
Nuts
Shellfish
Sea foods

FOODS HIGH IN MAGNESIUM

Raw tomatoes
Raw carrots
Roasted poultry
Roasted nuts
Unprocessed whole wheat
Boiled spinach
Cashew nuts
Citrus fruits
Fresh peas
Codfish
Brazil nuts
Brown rice
Peas, beans, and lentils

Hazelnuts
Oatmeal
Peaches
Peanuts
Pecans
Potatoes
Soy flour
Walnuts
Almonds
Barley
Halibut
Beef
Corn

FOODS HIGH IN MANGANESE

Unprocessed whole wheat
  flour
Whole grain rye
Sweet potatoes
Snap beans
Whole corn
Liver

Oatmeal
Wheat
Spinach
Beets
Lettuce
Kale
Dry beans

FOODS HIGH IN POTASSIUM

Buttermilk
Swiss cheese
Cow's milk
Goat's milk
Dried whey
Blackberries

Blueberries
Red currants
Red raspberries
Dried apricots
Brussels sprouts
Dandelion greens

Mustard greens
Turnip greens
Raw, dry beans
Brewer's yeast
Bran flakes
Dark rye flour
Cauliflower
Roasted nuts
Cooked meats
Seafoods
Chicken
All citrus fruits and juices
Dried dates, figs, and fruits
Prunes and raisins
Raw beets
Raw carrots
Raw parsnips
Raw potatoes
Radishes
Raw turnips
Asparagus

Beet greens
Raw cabbage
Endive
Avocados
Kale
Bananas
Cherries
Parsley
Spinach
Artichokes
Wild rice
Broccoli
Okra
Wheat germ
Rye wafers
Sweet corn
Lentils
Peas
Pumpkins
Soybeans
Tomato catsup

FOODS HIGH IN SODIUM

Cheddar cheese
Low fat cottage cheese
French dressing
Pork sausage
Canned crab
Canned fish
Canned carrots
Canned asparagus
Canned sauerkraut
Canned spinach
Tomato catsup
Chipped beef
Frankfurters
Cream cheese
Canned baked beans
Canned lima beans
Canned mushrooms
Dried cod

Rye bread
Butter
Buttermilk
Blue cheese
Margarine
Olives
Saltines
Bacon
Bologna
Cured ham
Liverwurst
Rye wafers
Unprocessed whole wheat
   flour
Salted nuts
Corned beef
Canned green peas

FOODS HIGH IN ZINC

Peanut butter
Canned pears
Canned cherries
Wheat bran
Beef liver
Oatmeal
Dry yeast
Whole corn
Pork liver
Cow's milk
Skim milk
Oysters
Canned applesauce

Peas
Eggs
Beef
Beets
Cabbage
Wheat
Barley
Spinach
Carrots
Clams
Herring
Lettuce

──────APPENDIX D──────

Organizations and Addresses

Note: The opinions expressed in this book do not necessarily reflect the views of any organization or affiliation of the authors.

Academy of Orthomolecular Psychiatry
1691 Northern Boulevard
Manhasset, NY 11030

American Academy of Medical Preventics
2811 "L" Street
Sacramento, CA 95816

Association for Chelation Therapy
P. O. Box 832
San Gabriel, CA 91775

Committee for Freedom of Choice in Cancer Therapy, Inc.
146 Main Street, #408
Los Altos, CA 94022

International Academy of Metabology
1000 East Walnut Street
Pasadena, CA 91106

International Academy of Preventive Medicine
10409 Town and Country Way, Suite 200
Houston, TX 77024

International College of Applied Nutrition
P. O. Box 386
La Habra, CA 90631

National Health Federation
212 West Foothill Boulevard
P. O. Box 688
Monrovia, CA 91016

Suggested Reading

Abrahamson, E. M., M.D., and A. W. Pezet, *Body, Mind and Sugar,* New York, Holt, Rinehart & Winston, 1951.

Brennan, R. O., with William C. Mulligan, *Nutrigenetics,* New York, M. Evans & Co., 1975.

Cheraskin, E., M.D., and W. M. Ringsdorf, Jr., M.D., with Arline Brecher, *New Hope for Incurable Diseases,* Hicksville, N.Y., Exposition Press, 1971.

———, *Psychodietetics,* New York, Bantam Books, 1974.

Culbert, Michael L., *Vitamin B17: Forbidden Weapon Against Cancer,* New Rochelle, N.Y., Arlington House, 1974.

———, *Freedom from Cancer,* Seal Beach, California, '76 Press and Committee for Freedom of Choice in Cancer Therapy, Inc., 1976.

Dufty, William, *Sugar Blues,* Radnor, Pa., Chilton Book Co., 1975.

Fredericks, Carlton, Ph.D., *Breast Cancer and the Nutritional Approach,* New York, Grosset and Dunlap, 1977.

———, *Eating Right for You,* New York, Grosset and Dunlap, 1972.

———, *PsychoNutrition,* New York, Grosset and Dunlap, 1976.

———, and Herman Goodman, M.D., *Low Blood Sugar and You,* New York, Grosset and Dunlap, 1969.

Fredman, Steven, M.D., and Robert Burger, *Forbidden Cures,* New York, Stein and Day, 1976.

Galton, Lawrence, *The Silent Disease: Hypertension,* New York, Crown Publishers, 1973.

Hoffer, Abram, M.D., Humphry Osmond, *How to Live with Schizophrenia,* New York, University Books, 1969.

Hur, Robin, *Food Reform: Our Desperate Need,* Austin, Texas, Heidelberg Publishers, 1975.

Kugler, Hans, Ph.D., *Doctor Kugler's Seven Keys to a Longer Life,* New York, Stein and Day, 1977.

Longgood, William, *The Poisons in Your Food,* New York, Pyramid Books, 1960.

Millman, Marcia, *The Unkindest Cut,* New York, Morrow and Co., 1977.

Nutrition Almanac, New York, McGraw-Hill Book Co., 1975.

Passwater, Richard A., *Supernutrition,* New York, Dial Press, 1975.
————, *Supernutrition for Healthy Hearts,* New York, Dial Press, 1977.
Pfeiffer, Carl, Ph.D., M.D., *Mental and Elemental Nutrients,* New Canaan, Conn., Keats Publishing, 1975.
Roberts, Sam E., M.D., *Exhaustion: Causes and Treatment,* Emmaus, Pa., Rodale Press, 1971.
Rosenberg, Harold, M.D., with A. N. Feldzamen, Ph.D., *The Doctor's Book of Vitamin Therapy,* New York, Berkley Windhover Books, 1974.
Williams, Roger J., Ph.D., D.Sc., *Alcoholism: The Nutritional Approach,* Austin, Tex., University of Texas Press, 1959.
————, *Nutrition Against Disease,* Bantam Books, New York, 1971.
————, *Physicians' Handbook of Nutritional Science,* Springfield, Ill., Charles C. Thomas, 1975.
Yudkin, John, M.D., *Sweet and Dangerous,* New York, Bantam Books, 1972.

Selected Bibliography

Abrahamson, E. M., M.D., and A. W. Pezet, *Body, Mind and Sugar,* New York, Holt, Rinehart & Winston, 1951.

Anatomy of a Coverup, Committee for Freedom of Choice in Cancer Therapy, Inc., Los Altos, Calif., 1975.

Barnes, Broda O., Ph.D., M.D., and Charlotte W. Barnes, M.A., *Heart Attack Rareness In Thyroid-Treated Patients,* Springfield, Ill., Charles C. Thomas, 1972.

Bealle, Morris A., *Super Drug Story,* Washington, D.C., Columbia Books, Inc., 1962.

Beard, John, *The Enzyme Treatment of Cancer and Its Scientific Basis,* London, Chatto and Windus, 1911.

Berman, Edgar, M.D., *The Solid Gold Stethoscope,* New York, Macmillan Publishing Co., Inc., 1976.

Blumer, W. and T. H. Reich, "Leaded Gasoline and Cancer Mortality," *Schweiz Med Wochenschr,* 106 (15): 503–6 (April 10, 1976).

Bolen, Jean Shinoda, "Meditation and Psychotherapy in the Treatment of Cancer," *Psychic,* August, 1973.

Brennan, R. O., with William C. Mulligan, *Nutrigenetics,* New York, M. Evans & Co., 1975.

Brewer, A. Keith and Richard Passwater, "Physics of the Cell Membrane; Mechanisms Involved in Cancer," Part V, *American Laboratory,* April, 1976.

Burk, Dean, Ph.D., *A Brief on Foods and Vitamins,* Sausalito, Calif., McNaughton Foundation, 1975.

———, Letter to Frank Rauscher, Jr., director, National Cancer Institute, April 20, 1973.

———, Letter to Rep. Louis Frey, Jr., May 30, 1972, *Cancer Control Journal,* May-June, 1973.

———, Letter to Rep. Robert A. Roe, July 3, 1973.

Cerami, Anthony and Charles M. Peterson, "Cyanate and Sickle-Cell Disease," *Scientific American,* April, 1975.

Cheraskin, E., M.D., and W. M. Ringsdorf, Jr., M.D., with Arline

Brecher, *New Hope for Incurable Diseases,* Hicksville, N.Y., Exposition Press, 1971.

———, *Psychodietetics,* New York, Bantam Books, 1974.

Contreras, Dr. Ernesto, *Reporte Preliminar; Comprendido de Pacientes Tratados con Laetrile-Amigdalina,* Tijuana, Mexico, 1967.

Culbert, Michael L., *Vitamin B17: Forbidden Weapon Against Cancer,* New Rochelle, N.Y., Arlington House, 1974.

———, *Freedom From Cancer,* Seal Beach, Calif., '76 Press and Committee for Freedom of Choice in Cancer Therapy, Inc., 1976.

Culliton, Barbara J., "Sloan-Kettering: The Trials of an Apricot Pit—1973," *Science,* December 1, 1973.

Dailey, J. E., and P. M. Marcuse, "Gonadotropin Secreting Giant Cell Carcinoma of the Lung." *Cancer* 24: 388–96 (August, 1969).

Danowski, T. S., M.D., *Diabetes As A Way of Life,* New York, Coward, McCann & Geoghegan, 1957.

Dayton, Seymour, "Nutrition and Atherosclerosis," *Progress in Food and Nutrition Science,* vol. 1, no. 3, pp. 191–206 (1975).

Dufty, William, *Sugar Blues,* Radnor, Pa., Chilton Book Co., 1975.

Ebel, Alfred, M.D., and John C. Kuo, M.D., "Tolerance for Treadmill Walking as an Index of Intermittent Claudition," *Archives of Physical Medicine and Rehabilitation,* vol. 48 (November, 1967).

Eckstein, Richard W., M.D., "Effect of Exercise and Coronary Artery Narrowing on Coronary Collateral Circulation," *Circulation Research,* vol. V (May, 1957).

Felland, Barbara, M.D., *Reprints of World's Literature on Minerals,* 3 vols.

Finestone, Albert J., M.D., and Michael G. Wohl, M.D., "Hypoglycemia: A Complex Problem," *Medical Clinics of North America,* vol. 54, no. 2 (March, 1970).

"Food for Life," *Town & Country,* April and May, 1976.

Frank, Charles W., M.D., Eve Weinblatt, Sam Shapiro, and Robert V. Sager, M.D., "Physical Inactivity as a Lethal Factor in Myocardial Infarction among Men," *Circulation,* vol. 34 (December, 1966).

Fredericks, Carlton, Ph.D., *Breast Cancer and the Nutritional Approach,* New York, Grosset and Dunlap, 1977.

———, *Eating Right for You,* New York, Grosset and Dunlap, 1972.

———, *PsychoNutrition,* New York, Grosset and Dunlap, 1976.

———, and Herman Goodman, M.D., *Low Blood Sugar and You,* New York, Grosset and Dunlap, 1969.

Fredman, Steven, M.D., and Robert Burger, *Forbidden Cures,* New York, Stein and Day, 1976.

Freikel, Norbert, M.D. *et al.,* "Alcohol Hypoglycemia," *Diabetes,* vol. 14, no. 6.

Galton, Lawrence, *The Silent Disease: Hypertension,* New York, Crown Publishers, 1973.

Gordon, Garry, M.D., and Robert Vance, D.O., "EDTA Chelation Therapy for Arteriosclerosis: History and Mechanisms of Action," *Osteopathic Annals*, vol. 4, no. 2 (February, 1976).

Griffin, G. Edward, *World Without Cancer*, American Media, 1974.

Guidetti, Ettore, "Observations Preliminaires sur Quelques Cas de Cancer Traites par un Glycuronoside Cyanogenetique," *Acta Unio Internationalis Contra Cancrum* 11:156–58 (1955).

Gurchot, Charles, *Biology—The Key to the Riddle of Cancer*, New York, Moore Publishers, 1949.

———, "The Trophoblast Theory of Cancer (John Beard, 1857–1924) Revisited," *Oncology*, vol. 31, no. 5-6 (1975).

Harper, Harold W., M.D., and Garry Gordon, M.D., eds., *Reprints of Medical Literature on Chelation Therapy*, Sacramento, Calif., American Academy of Medical Preventics.

Hoffer, Abram, M.D., Humphry Osmond, *How to Live with Schizophrenia*, New York, University Books, 1969.

Hur, Robin, *Food Reform: Our Desperate Need*, Austin, Texas, Heidelberg Publishers, 1975.

Illingworth, Barbara, Ph.D., "Enzymatic Defects as Causes of Hypoglycemia," *Diabetes*, vol. 14 (June, 1965).

Jones, Stewart M., M.D., *The Immoral Banning of Vitamin B-17: How It Came About an How It Is Continuing*, privately published, Palo Alto, Calif., 1974.

———, *Nutrition Rudiments in Cancer*, privately published, Palo Alto, Calif., 1972.

Kahn, Harold A., "Change in Serum Cholesterol Associated with Changes in the United States Civilian Diet, 1909–1965," *The American Journal of Clinical Nutrition*, vol. 23, no. 7:879–882 (July, 1970).

Kannel, William B., M.D. *et al.*, "Intermittent Claudication," *Circulation*, vol. 41 (May, 1970).

Kittler, Glenn D., *Laetrile—Control for Cancer*, New York, Paperback Library, 1963.

Koobs, D. H., "Phosphate Mediation of the Crabtree and Pasteur Effects," *Science*, October 17, 1972.

Krebs, Ernst T., Jr., "The Nitrilosides in Plants and Animals," *The Laetriles—Nitrilosides—in the Prevention and Control of Cancer*, McNaughton Foundation, Sausalito, Calif., 1967.

———, "The Nitrilosides (Vitamin B-17)—Their Nature, Occurrence and Metabolic Significance," *Journal of Applied Nutrition* 22, nos. 3 and 4 (1970).

———, and N. R. Bouziane, "Nitrilosides (Laetriles)," *The Laetriles—Nitrilosides—in the Prevention and Control of Cancer*, McNaughton Foundation, Sausalito, Calif., 1967.

———, Ernst T. Krebs, Sr., and Howard H. Beard, "The Unitarian or Trophoblastic Thesis of Cancer," *Medical Record*, July, 1950.

Kugler, Hans, Ph.D., *Doctor Kugler's Seven Keys to a Longer Life*, New York, Stein and Day, 1977.

Kuo, Peter T., M.D., and Claude R. Joyner, M.D., "Angina Pectoris Induced by Rat Ingestion in Patients with Coronary Artery Disease," *Journal of the American Medical Association*, July 23, 1955.

Kupers, Edward C., M.D., "Feeding the Elderly Heart," *American Geriatrics Society*, vol. 22, no. 3 (March, 1974).

"Laetrile—An Answer to Cancer?" *Prevention*, December, 1971.

Larson, Gena, "Is There an Anti-Cancer Food?" *Prevention*, April, 1972.

Lea, Koch, Morris, "Tumor-Selective Inhibition of Incorporation of 3H-Labeled Amino Acids into Protein by Cyanate," *Cancer Research*, September 1975.

Longgood, William, *The Poisons in Your Food*, New York, Pyramid Books, 1960.

Matchan, Don C., "A New Look at Laetrile," *Let's Live*, June, 1973.

McCarty, Mark, "Burying Caesar: An Analysis of the Laetrile Problem," *Triton Times*, University of California at San Diego, November 29, 1975.

Miller, Benjamin F., M.D., and Lawrence Galton, with Daniel Brunner, M.D., *Freedom from Heart Attacks*, New York, Simon & Schuster, 1972.

Morrone, John A., "Chemotherapy of Inoperable Cancer (Preliminary Report of 10 Cases Treated with Laetrile)," *Experimental Medicine and Surgery* 4 (1962).

Navarro, Manuel D., "Biochemistry of Laetrile Therapy in Cancer," *Papyrus* 1:8–9, 27–28 (1957).

———, "Early Cancer Detection," *Journal of the Philippine Medical Association* 36:425–32 (1960); and "Early Cancer Detection—A Biochemical Approach," *Santo Tomás Journal of Medicine* 15: 111–29 (1960).

———, "Laetrile in Malignancy," *Santo Tomás Journal of Medicine* 10 (1955).

———, "Laetrile—The Ideal Anti-Cancer Drug?" *Santo Tomás Journal of Medicine* 9:468–71 (1954).

———, "Mechanism of Action and Therapeutic Effects of Laetrile in Cancer," *Journal of the Philippine Medical Association* 33:620–27 (1957).

———, "Why Are Cancer Patients 'Pregnant'?" *Santo Tomás Journal of Medicine* 26, no. 3 (1971).

Pagliara, Anthony S., M.D. *et al.*, "Hypoglycemia in Infancy and Childhood," Parts I and II, *Journal of Pediatrics*, vol. 82, no. 3, pp. 365–79.

Passwater, Richard A., *Supernutrition*, New York, Dial Press, 1975.

————, *Supernutrition for Healthy Hearts,* New York, Dial Press, 1977.

Pfeiffer, Carl, Ph.D., M.D., *Mental and Elemental Nutrients,* New Canaan. Conn., Keats Publishing, 1975.

Physician's Handbook of Vitamin B-17 Therapy, McNaughton Foundation, Science Press International, Sausalito, Calif., 1973.

Reitnauer, P. G., "Prolongation of Life in Tumor-Bearing Mice by Bitter Almonds," *Arch. Geschwulstforsch,* 42, no. 4, pp. 135–37 (East Germany, 1974).

A Report on the Treatment of Cancer with Beta-Cyanogenetic Glucosides ('Laetriles')," California Department of Public Health (California Cancer Advisory Council), May, 1963.

Roberts, Sam E., M.D., *Exhaustion: Causes and Treatment,* Emmaus, Pa., Rodale Press. 1971.

Rosenberg, Harold, M.D., with A. N. Feldzamen, Ph.D., *The Doctor's Book of Vitamin Therapy,* New York, Berkley Windhover Books, 1974.

Ross, R. S., "Ischemic Heart Disease: An Overview," *American Journal of Cardiology* 36: 495–505 (October, 1975).

Ross, Walter S., "The Medicines We Need—But Can't Have," *Reader's Digest.* October, 1973.

Schroeder, Henry, M.D., *The Trace Elements and Man,* Old Greenwich, Conn., Devin-Adair Co., 1973.

Seven, M. J., M.D., ed., *Metal Binding in Medicine,* Philadelphia, J. B. Lippincott Company, 1960.

Shute, Wilfred E., M.D., *Dr. Wilfred Shute's Complete Updated Vitamin E Book,* New Canaan. Conn., Keats Publishing, 1975.

Singer, Adolf, M.B., and Charles Rob, M.C., "The Fate of the Claudicator," *British Medical Journal,* vol. 2, pp. 633–36 (August 27, 1960).

Soffer, A., *Chelation Therapy,* Springfield, Ill., Charles C. Thomas Publishers, 1964.

Stang, Alan, "Laetrile: Freedom of Choice in Cancer Therapy?" *American Opinion,* January, 1974.

Stefansson, Vilhjalmur, *Cancer: Disease of Civilization,* New York, Hill & Wang, 1960.

Stone, Daniel B., M.B. and William Connor, M.D., "The Prolonged Effects of a Low Cholesterol, High Carbohydrate Diet upon the Serum Lipids in Diabetic Patients," *Diabetes,* vol. 12 (March-April, 1963).

Summa, Herbert, M., "Amygdalin, A Physiologically Active Therapeutic Agent in Malignancies," *Krebsgeschehen* 4 (West Germany, 1972).

Summary of the McNaughton Foundation IND 6734 (April 6, 1970– February, 1971), *Recent Case Histories [and] the "Grandfather-*

ing" of Laetrile-Amygdalin in the Treatment of Cancer, McNaughton Foundation, Sausalito, Calif., 1973.

Tasca, Marco, "Observazioni Cliniche Sugli Effetti Terapeutici ci un Glicuronoside cianogenetico in Casi di Neoplasie Maligne Umane," *Gazzetta Medica Italiana,* Edizioni Minerva Medica (1958).

Taylor, Henry Longstree, Ph.D. *et al.,* "Death Rates Among Physically Active and Sedentary Employees of the Railroad Industry," *American Journal of Public Health,* October, 1962, pp. 1697–707.

Taylor, Renee, *Hunza Health Secrets,* New York, Award Books, 1969.

Tripathy, Kshetrabasi, M.D., Hernan Lotero, M.D., and Oscar Bolanos, M.D., "Role of Dietary Protein upon Serum Cholesterol Level in Malnourished Subjects," *The American Journal of Clinical Nutrition,* vol. 23, no. 9, pp. 1160–68 (September, 1970).

Voors, A. W., M. S. Shuman, and P. N. Gallagher, "Atherosclerosis and Hypertension in Relation to Some Trace Elements in Tissues," *World Review of Nutrition and Dietetics,* vol. 20, pp. 299–326.

West, Kelly M., M.D. and John M. Kalbfleisch, M.D., "Influence of Nutritional Factors on Prevalence of Diabetes," *Diabetes,* vol. 20, no. 1, pp. 99–108.

Whichelow, M. J., N.A. *et al.,* "Critical Analysis of Blood Sugar Measurements in Diabetes Detection and Diagnosis," *Diabetes,* vol. 16, no. 4, pp. 219–26.

Williams, Roger J., Ph.D., D.Sc., *Alcoholism: The Nutritional Approach,* Austin, Tex., University of Texas Press, 1959.

———, *Nutrition Against Disease,* New York, Bantam Books, 1971.

———, *Physicians' Handbook of Nutritional Science,* Springfield, Ill. Charles C. Thomas, 1975.

Yudkin, John, M.D., *Sweet and Dangerous,* New York, Bantam Books, 1972.

Index

PABA, 209
pain, cancer, 148, 168, 172, 173
Pangamic acid. *See* vitamin B₁₅
Panthothenic acid, 209
parathyroid glands, 102
Passwater, Richard, 152
Pauling, Linus, 129, 130, 170, 189
Pavlov, Alexander, 120
Pfeiffer, Carl, 80
phosphorus, 218
plaques, arteriosclerotic, 83–89
pollution, 30–46, 49, 75, 87, 91, 119, 131, 132, 145, 146, 147, 153, 160, 162, 169, 171, 188, 192, 193, 194, 197
potassium, 48, 184, 193, 194, 218, 222–23
preservatives. *See* food preservatives
Privitera, James, 138
protein drink, 76, 187, 202
protein, predigested, 168
Proxmire, William, 41
prudent diet, 124, 179
Psychodietetics, 186

Qolla Indians, 59

radiation, 115, 122, 123, 128, 139, 153, 161, 167
Rauscher, Frank, Jr., 117
retinoids, 130–31
Richardson, John A., 137–38
Ross, R. S., 98
Roswell Park Memorial Institute for Cancer Research, 117
Rubin, David, 159
Rutherford, Glen, 133–34, 139

salt, 185–86, 194
schizophrenia, 58
Schlegel, Jorgen, 130

Seifter, Eli, 130
selenium, 102, 152, 170, 219
Senate Health Subcommittee, 144
Senate Select Committee on Nutrition, 127, 185
Seventh-Day Adventists, 125, 158
sickle-cell anemia, 147
Simonton, O. Carl, 26, 164–66
Sloan-Kettering Cancer Center. *See* Memorial Sloan-Kettering Cancer Center
smoking, 74, 112, 125, 153, 160, 168, 180, 194
sodium, 184, 193–94, 219, 223
sodium nitrate, 36, 119
The Solid Gold Stethoscope, 52, 95, 121
Soto, Mario, 140
Spokane, Washington, approach to vascular catastrophes, 95–96
Stare, Frederick, 40
Stone, Irwin, 129, 130, 170, 189
stress, 45–46, 48, 54, 87, 110, 132
stroke, 89, 92, 93, 185
sugar, 25, 34–38, 59, 65, 71, 74, 77, 127, 131, 168, 180, 185–86
Sugiura, Kanematso, 141–43
Supernutrition, 152
surgery, 19, 115, 128, 139, 161, 167, 196. *See also* bypass surgery

Temin, Howard, 117
Thalidomide, 43
thermography, 107–109
Thomas, Caroline Bedell, 163
transfer factor, 131
triglycerides, 100
trophoblast, 147, 153–56, 158, 160–61, 164, 169, 178
tumefactions, 123

239